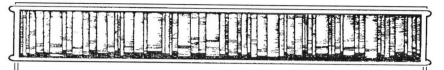

Robert S. Galen, MD, MPH, FASCP
*Professor and Head, Department
of Health Administration,
College of Public Health,
University of Georgia,
Athens*

Jack E. Fincham, PhD

Patient Compliance with Medications
Issues and Opportunities

NOTES FOR PROFESSIONAL LIBRARIANS AND LIBRARY USERS

This is an original book title published by Pharmaceutical Products Press®, An Imprint of The Haworth Press, Inc. Unless otherwise noted in specific chapters with attribution, materials in this book have not been previously published elsewhere in any format or language.

CONSERVATION AND PRESERVATION NOTES

All books published by The Haworth Press, Inc., and its imprints are printed on certified pH neutral, acid-free book grade paper. This paper meets the minimum requirements of American National Standard for Information Sciences-Permanence of Paper for Printed Material, ANSI Z39.48-1984.

DIGITAL OBJECT IDENTIFIER (DOI) LINKING

The Haworth Press is participating in reference linking for elements of our original books. (For more information on reference linking initiatives, please consult the CrossRef Web site at www.crossref.org.) When citing an element of this book such as a chapter, include the element's Digital Object Identifier (DOI) as the last item of the reference. A Digital Object Identifier is a persistent, authoritative, and unique identifier that a publisher assigns to each element of a book. Because of its persistence, DOIs will enable The Haworth Press and other publishers to link to the element referenced, and the link will not break over time. This will be a great resource in scholarly research.

Patient Compliance with Medications

Issues and Opportunities

PHARMACEUTICAL PRODUCTS PRESS®
Titles of Related Interest

Pharmacy Ethics edited by Mickey Smith, Steven Strauss, H. John Baldwin, and Kelly T. Alberts

Advancing Prescription Medicine Compliance: New Paradigms, New Practices edited by Jack E. Fincham

A History of Nonprescription Product Regulation by W. Steven Pray

Pharmacy and the U.S. Health Care System, Third Edition edited by Michael Ira Smith, Albert I. Wertheimer, and Jack E. Fincham

Taking Your Medicine: A Guide to Medication Regimens and Compliance for Patients and Caregivers by Jack E. Fincham

Patient Compliance with Medications
Issues and Opportunities

Jack E. Fincham, PhD

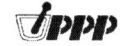

Pharmaceutical Products Press®
An Imprint of The Haworth Press, Inc.
New York

For more information on this book or to order, visit
http://www.haworthpress.com/store/product.asp?sku=5365

or call 1-800-HAWORTH (800-429-6784) in the United States and Canada
or (607) 722-5857 outside the United States and Canada
or contact orders@HaworthPress.com

Published by

Pharmaceutical Products Press®, an imprint of The Haworth Press, Inc., 10 Alice Street, Binghamton, NY 13904-1580.

PUBLISHER'S NOTE

The development, preparation, and publication of this work has been undertaken with great care. However, the Publisher, employees, editors, and agents of The Haworth Press are not responsible for any errors contained herein or for consequences that may ensue from use of materials or information contained in this work. The Haworth Press is committed to the dissemination of ideas and information according to the highest standards of intellectual freedom and the free exchange of ideas. Statements made and opinions expressed in this publication do not necessarily reflect the views of the Publisher, Directors, management, or staff of The Haworth Press, Inc., or an endorsement by them.

This book has been published solely for educational purposes and is not intended to substitute for the medical advice of a treating physician. Medicine is an ever-changing science. As new research and clinical experience broaden our knowledge, changes in treatment may be required. While many potential treatment options are made herein, some or all of the options may not be applicable to a particular individual. Therefore, the author, editor and publisher do not accept responsibility in the event of negative consequences incurred as a result of the information presented in this book. We do not claim that this information is necessarily accurate by the rigid scientific and regulatory standards applied for medical treatment. **No warranty, express or implied, is furnished with respect to the material contained in this book. The reader is urged to consult with his/her personal physician with respect to the treatment of any medical condition.**

Cover design by Lora Wiggins.

Library of Congress Cataloging-in-Publication Data

Patient compliance with medications: issues and opportunities/Jack E. Fincham, editor.
   p. cm.
   Includes bibliographical references and index.
   ISBN: 978-0-7890-2609-5 (hard : alk. paper)
   ISBN: 978-0-7890-2610-1 (soft : alk. paper)
   1. Drugs—Administration. 2. Patient compliance. I. Fincham, Jack E. [DNLM: 1. Drug Therapy. 2. Patient Compliance. 3. Physician's Role. 4. Treatment Refusal. WB 330 P298 2007]
RM147.P38 2007
615.5′8—dc22
                                                                      2006034985

This book is dedicated to Ms. Meg and Mr. Morteau—
there are none finer than these two.

CONTENTS

ABOUT THE AUTHOR

Dr. Jack E. Fincham is a graduate of the University of Nebraska College of Pharmacy and was a Kellogg Pharmaceutical Clinical Scientist Fellow at the University of Minnesota where he obtained his PhD in Social and Administrative Pharmacy. Dr. Fincham has completed a Post Graduate Certificate Degree in Health Economics at the University of Aberdeen, Scotland. Dr. Fincham has held academic, research, and administrative positions at several Schools and Colleges of Pharmacy. He has researched varying topics pertaining to patient compliance, medication management, the Medicare drug benefit, smoking cessation, and health economics. Dr. Fincham currently serves as the A. W. Jowdy Professor of Pharmacy Care at the UGA College of Pharmacy and Professor of Public Health in the UGA College of Public Health. He is a member of the University of Georgia Teaching Academy. From 1994 to 2004, Dr. Fincham served as dean of the University of Kansas School of Pharmacy.

Dr. Fincham has authored over 200 refereed and professional manuscripts published in sixty journals. He has made over 200 professional and research presentations to allied health, dental, medical, information technology, nursing, nutrition, pharmacy, and public health professional groups from Vietnam, China, Asia, Australia, Canada, Europe, the United Kingdom, and the United States. He has edited and written ten books. Dr. Fincham is the founding editor of the *Journal of Public Health Pharmacy* and serves as the associate editor of the *American Journal of Pharmaceutical Education*. Dr. Fincham authored *Taking Your Medicine: A Guide to Medication Regimens and Compliance for Patients and Caregivers,* published by The Haworth Press (www.takingyourmedicine.com). This book has been listed as one of the "Best consumer health books of 2005" by *Library Journal*. He has recently completed the book: *The Medicare*

Patient Compliance with Medications: Issues and Opportunities
© 2007 by The Haworth Press, Inc. All rights reserved.
doi:10.1300/5365_a

Part D Program: Making the Most of the Benefit, published by Jones & Bartlett Publishers.

Dr. Fincham is an active member of numerous pharmacy, public health, and academic associations. He currently serves as a member of the Nonprescription Drug Advisory Committee of the U.S. Food and Drug Administration and has served as an advisor for the CMS Medicare Drug Benefit Program from 2003 until 2007. Dr. Fincham is a Fellow in the American Society of Consultant Pharmacists, a member of Phi Beta Delta Honor Society for International Scholars, Phi Kappa Phi Honor Society, the Rho Chi Pharmaceutical Honor Society, and the Phi Lambda Sigma Pharmacy Leadership Society. In 1997, he was named the recipient of the Faculty Excellence in Pharmacy Administration Award by the National Community Pharmacists Association. Also in 1997, he was given the Dean's Award for Sustained Contributions to Community Pharmacy Practice by the American College of Apothecaries. In 1998, he was listed as one of the top fifty most influential pharmacists in the United States by *Drug Topics* magazine.

CONTRIBUTORS

Christopher L. Cook, PharmD, PhD, is a clinical assistant professor in the department of clinical and administrative pharmacy at the University of Georgia College of Pharmacy. Dr. Cook's specialty areas include diabetes mellitus, patient compliance, and provision of pharmaceutical care to patients in varying settings.

Jenny Gowan, PhD, Grad Dip Comm Pharm, PhC, FACPP, FPS, AACPA, MSHPA, is an accredited consultant pharmacist promoting quality use of medicines at the Northern and North Eastern Divisions of General Practice in Melbourne, Australia. She is a special lecturer in the Department of Pharmacy Practice, Monash University. She has developed and presented many continuing professional education programs throughout Australia including the "One Minute Counsellor," "Multiple Medication Management," and Therapeutic Update courses. She, together with Dr. Louis Roller, writes a counseling and medication review article each month for the *Australian Journal of Pharmacy.* Dr. Gowan works as a practicing community pharmacist and carries out many medication reviews in residential and domiciliary settings.

Louis Roller, PhD, MSc, BSc, DipEd, BPharm, FPS, FACPP, is the associate dean of teaching, Victorian College of Pharmacy, Monash University, and a member of the Department of Pharmacy Practice. He is also a senior associate of the medical faculty at the University of Melbourne. He has been involved in continuing pharmacy education in Victoria for four decades and has also lectured regularly interstate and overseas. He is a member of the Pharmacy Board of Victoria and is currently chairman of the Education Committee of the board. He is on the editorial boards of two international journals of pharmacy practice and has published widely in the area of pharmacy practice in-

Patient Compliance with Medications: Issues and Opportunities
© 2007 by The Haworth Press, Inc. All rights reserved.
doi:10.1300/5365_b

cluding over 120 medication management case studies with Dr. Jenny Gowan in the *Australian Journal of Pharmacy*. Dr. Gowan and Dr. Roller are the authors of the highly successful book titled *Practical Disease State Management for Pharmacists,* Australian Pharmaceutical Publishing Company Limited, Melbourne, Australia, 2004.

Jayashri Sankaranarayanan, PhD, is an assistant professor of pharmacy practice at the University of Nebraska Medical Center College of Pharmacy. Dr. Sankaranarayanan's research interests include patient self-management readiness and behavior adherence related to chronic disease management, and expanding the role and quality of pharmacy services.

Richard Schulz, PhD, is a professor of pharmaceutical and health outcomes sciences at the University of South Carolina College of Pharmacy, and an adjunct professor at the Norman J. Arnold School of Public Health, University of South Carolina. His areas of expertise include pharmacoepidemiology, quality of life assessment, patient behavior regarding prescription medication, and mental health topics and applications.

Chapter 1

Introduction

Illness is the night-side of life, a more onerous citizenship. Everyone who is born holds dual citizenship, in the kingdom of the well and in the kingdom of the sick. Although we all prefer to use only the good passport, sooner or later each of us is obliged, at least for a spell, to identify ourselves as citizens of that other place.

Susan Sontag, *Illness As Metaphor* (1977)

Illness is often difficult for all of us, and usually the response to illness is individual specific. Most patients are willing to do all that is possible to obtain an optimum health status. For those that wish to get well or stay well, patient compliance can enhance the potential patients have to achieve health objectives and goals. Patients face a bewildering array of challenges in the health care system, their health conditions, and necessary actions to obtain or maintain optimal health. Illness affects many; no one is spared in one way or another.

One necessary requirement for many for obtaining a better state of health is the taking of a prescribed or an over-the-counter (OTC) medication for treatment purposes. The use of drugs as a form of medical treatment in the United States is an enormously complex process. Individuals can purchase medications through numerous outlets. Over-the-counter (OTC) medications can be purchased in pharmacies, grocery stores, supermarkets, convenience stores, via the Internet, and through any number of additional outlets. Prescriptions can be purchased through traditional channels (community chain and

Patient Compliance with Medications: Issues and Opportunities
© 2007 by The Haworth Press, Inc. All rights reserved.
doi:10.1300/5365_01

independent pharmacies), from mail service pharmacies, through the Internet, from physicians, from health care institutions, and from elsewhere. The monitoring of the positive and negative outcomes of the use of these drugs, both prescription and OTC, can be disjointed and incomplete.

External variables may greatly influence patients and their drug-taking behaviors. Coverage for prescribed drugs allows those with coverage to obtain medications with varying cost-sharing requirements. However, many do not have insurance coverage for drugs or other health-related needs. It has been estimated that for the two-year period between 2002 and 2003, 44.7 million individuals (18 percent of the population) under the age of 65 were without health insurance (Kaiser Family Foundation, 2004; Miller, 2001). Certainly, these considerations have huge ramifications for how and when consumers obtain prescribed and OTC medications. Whether they have coverage or not for prescription drugs, patients may choose to be noncompliant. It is much more complex than just consideration of insurance coverage.

Everyone talks about it, all benefit from it, and no one knows as much as what is necessary about patient compliance. Compliance, or lack thereof, affects us all. One of the most understated problems in the delivery of health care services is patient noncompliance, its occurrence, impacts upon it, and associated outcomes if allowed to continue without intervention. Health professionals need to see influencing patient compliance as a required role obligation. The goal of the text will be to present means for health professionals to assume ownership of the issue of noncompliance with medications for the patients for whom they provide care.

This book seeks to explore compliance behavior, impacts (positive or negative) upon it, and opportunities that exist for influencing noncompliant behavior. Thus the issue of noncompliance will be explored with the intent of examining opportunities for improvement and maintenance of compliant behavior with prescribed drugs.

The issues related to compliance will not be solved with the publication of this book. Only through the empowering of patients, and working with those who are not optimally compliance, will success be achieved. The reality of the situations is such that the problems of patient noncompliance must be solved one patient at a time.

REFERENCES

Kaiser Family Foundation (2004). The uninsured and their access to health care. Washington, DC: Fact sheet #1420-06, November, 2004.

Miller, J. L. (2001). A perfect storm: The confluence of forces affecting health care coverage. Washington, DC: National Coalition on Health Care.

Santag, S. (1977). *Illness As Metaphor* New York: Farrar, Straus and Giroux.

Chapter 2

Scope of Noncompliance
and Other Issues

Patient compliance with medications and regimens is a part of the process of drug use by patients. The prescribed drugs that patients take can be a small part of total drug use by patients. Other drugs taken may include over-the-counter (OTC) drugs, herbal supplements, vitamins, nutritional supplements, and perhaps drugs borrowed from other friends, family members, or perfect strangers. This book relates to compliance and patients, and how to improve the former for the benefit of the latter. However, it is important to consider other aspects of drug use, both prescription and other types of drugs. Elsewhere in this book, specifics about health professionals and impacts upon patient compliance will be presented; pharmacists and their role in compliance are discussed in this chapter.

DRUGS, PHARMACISTS, AND INSURANCE

Drugs As a Form of Treatment

The use of drugs as a form of medical treatment in the United States is an enormously complex process. Individuals can purchase medications through numerous outlets. Over-the-counter (OTC) medications can be purchased in pharmacies, grocery stores, supermarkets, convenience stores, via the Internet, and through any number of additional outlets. Prescriptions can be purchased through traditional channels (community chain and independent pharmacies), from mail

Patient Compliance with Medications: Issues and Opportunities
© 2007 by The Haworth Press, Inc. All rights reserved.
doi:10.1300/5365_02

service pharmacies, through the Internet, from physicians, from health care institutions, and elsewhere. The monitoring of the positive and negative outcomes of the use of these drugs, both prescription and OTC, can be disjointed and incomplete.

Pharmacies and Pharmacists

It is important to realize that although pharmacists are the gatekeepers for patients to obtain prescription drugs, patients can obtain prescription medications from other pharmacies and/or from dispensing physicians. Patients may also borrow from friends, relatives, or even casual acquaintances. In addition, patients obtain OTC medications from physicians through prescriptions, on advice from pharmacists, through self-selection, or through the recommendations of friends or acquaintances. Through all of this, it must be recognized that there is a formal (structural) and informal (word of mouth) component at play. Pharmacists or physicians may or may not be consulted regarding the use of medications. But in some cases, health professionals are unaware of the drugs patients are taking. In addition, herbal remedies or health supplements may be taken without the knowledge or input of a health professional.

As an example, consider the patient medication profiling capability of most pharmacists. Computerization of patient medication records is commonplace in pharmacy. This computerization allows for ease in billing third-party prescription programs, maintenance of drug allergy information, allows for drug-use review, notification of drug interactions, and aids in the meeting of OBRA '90 requirements. Thus, computerization permits drug-related information to be easily entered, retained, and retrieved. However, OTC medications are rarely entered into such records (one exception may be OTC drugs prescribed by physicians and dispensed through a prescription by pharmacists). This exclusion of a whole class of drugs from the monitoring programs of pharmacy may have a profound effect upon the ability of pharmacists to monitor the drug therapies of their patients. If the patient purchases the OTC medication in the pharmacy, the pharmacist may have an idea of the drugs consumed. However, if the OTC drugs are purchased in a nonpharmacy outlet, the pharmacist is completely in the dark concerning many drugs a patient may be taking. Patients may also utilize numerous pharmacies for varying prescription products, in which case there is no one record repository for all medications patients may be taking.

Insurance Coverage or Lack Thereof

External variables may greatly influence patients and their drug-taking behaviors. Coverage for prescribed drugs allows those with coverage to obtain medications with varying cost-sharing requirements. However, many do not have insurance coverage for drugs or other health-related needs. It has been estimated that for the year, 2004, 14.7 percent of the U.S. population were without health insurance for all or part of this period (Family Core Component of the 1997-2004 National Health Interview Surveys, 2005). This amounts to slightly over 42 million Americans. Certainly, these considerations have huge ramifications for how and when consumers obtain prescribed and OTC medications. Those that do have health insurance have seen premiums rise drastically in the recent past, 8.4 percent in 2000, and 11 percent in 2001 (Miller, 2001). Miller (2001) notes that employees are not just being asked to pay more for health insurance, but to pay it all.

SELF-CARE

When examining the utilization of health care, the possibility exists that an individual strives to obtain an optimal state of health but yet does do not look to health care providers for advice regarding a health problem. Ory, DeFriese, and Duncker (1998) have suggested that self-care "has evolved in usage to identify a particular role for laypersons in shaping both the processes and outcomes of the care they receive from professionals, a role extending to the self-management of chronic conditions" (p. xv). Ory et al. (1998) also indicate that self-care involved actions persons take to self-diagnose and prevent or treat common conditions, both acute and chronic (pp. xvi-xvii).

Through self-care, an individual may enter the health care system only so far, perhaps to obtain a diagnosis, but will not rely on a physician for treatment of the diagnosed condition. Self-help or self-care may be utilized to try to treat the condition. Appropriateness of self-care lies in the ability of patients to interpret symptoms and understand the symptom experience and what it means (Stoller, Forster, & Portugal, 1993). Dean (1986) describes four components of self-directed care:

1. individual self-care;
2. family care;
3. care from extended social network; and
4. mutual aid responses to health problems, self-help groups.

Self-care can have tangible benefits for many involved in health care delivery. An active orientation toward health care can serve to foster a partnership between physician and patient. Self-limiting conditions could be treated by the individual as well as providers other than the physician, namely a pharmacist. Self-care could save the patient time and expense, and the need for more costly care could be averted.

Self-care or self-help may be one of the unrecognized causes or contributors to noncompliance with prescribed medical and therapeutic regiments. The individual patient may feel that, in the case of drugs, a certain medication may not be needed to treat a certain condition, or that a different medication other then the one prescribed would be more appropriate.

SELF-MEDICATION

Self-medication can be broadly defined as a decision made by a patient to consume a drug with or without the approval or direction of a health professional. The self-medication activities of patients have increased dramatically in the late twentieth century. Many current impacts upon patients have continued to fuel this increase. There are ever increasing locations from which to purchase OTC medications. There have been many prescription items switched to OTC classification in the last fifty years. In addition, patients are increasingly becoming comfortable with self-diagnosing and self-selection of OTC remedies. The number of switched products is dramatically and significantly fueling the rapid expansion of OTC drug usage (Gannon, 1991; Janoff, 1999). Dean (1996) notes that in many studies, self-medication with nonprescribed therapies exceeds the use of prescription medications.

These factors influencing self-medication in turn affect pharmacists. Certainly economically, as more OTC products are available for purchase, and in places in which to purchase them, pharmacists are affected. As self-diagnosis and self-selection of products occurs, pharmacists may not be fully aware of all drugs patients are taking.

Patients' use of self-selected products can have enormous potential benefits for patients, as well as for others (Catford, 1995). Through the rational use of drugs, patients may avoid more costly therapies or professional services. Self-limiting conditions on even some chronic health conditions (allergies, dermatological conditions, etc.), if appropriately treated through patient self-medication, allow the patient to have a degree of autonomy in health care decisions.

Advocates of self-medication have suggested that the patient properly educated to self-medicate are more likely to be independent, knowledgeable, and compliant (Kelly, 1994). Elsewhere, it has been suggested that patient self-medication is a form of patient education (Barry, 1993).

OTCs are widely used by all age groups. In a large cohort of preschool-age children, 53.7 percent of children had been given some type of OTC medication in the past thirty days (Kogan, Pappas, Yu, & Kotelchuck, 1994). The efficacy and effectiveness of OTCs use in children has been challenged. In a critical review of clinical trials over a forty-year period in preschool children, Smith and Feldman concluded that "no good evidence has demonstrated the effectiveness of OTC remedies" (Smith & Feldman, 1993). Elsewhere, Weiland (1996) points to the risks in which patients may be placed by OTC use.

The prominence of OTC usage will continue for several reasons. Manufacturers leverage OTCs when prescription-only products are more suitably made available for patient's self-use and when patent protection is lost on products that are generally safe for patients. Retailers appreciate the profitability of OTC products in their sales mix. Patients favor products easily purchased as OTCs and for which they do not need to be seen by a physician and receive a prescription for use in a self-medication situation. Pharmacists should not forget about this important classification of drugs when assessing patient profiles and examining appropriateness of other consumed products by patients, whether they be by prescription or OTC.

PATIENT COMPLIANCE ISSUES

The consequences and ramifications of patient noncompliance with medication regimens pervade all aspects of the delivery of health care. Noncompliance is potential by deleterious to pharmaceutical manufacturers, prescribers, dispensers, patients, and to society as a whole.

Whose Problem Is It?

Whose problem is noncompliance (Sbarbaro & Stener, 1991)? Some have questioned the treatments many patients receive and ask whether cooperation with, or control of patients is a goal (Kjellgren, Ahlner, & Saljo, 1995). Others argue about the term to use—compliance or adherence (Fawcett, 1995). Elliot (1994) has noted that adherence with medication parallels adherence with appointments (1994). Some patients are accidentally noncompliant (Isaac & Tamblyn, 1993) and simply do not realize their noncompliant behavior.

Role of the Pharmacist

Pharmacists can significantly impact upon patient noncompliance. It is not possible to entirely control the use of drugs by patients. Since drugs can be obtained from so many varied sources, the pharmacist is often unable to be fully aware of all locations where a patient obtains medications. However, pharmacists can play a major, active role in ensuring proper patient compliance. The role of the pharmacist as an optimizer of patient compliance cannot be overstated (Bruzek, 1994). Therapeutic benefits to patients, economic rewards to pharmacists, and more appropriate usage of health resources will all be enhanced through appropriate patient compliance monitoring by pharmacists.

How Can Pharmacists Impact Noncompliance?

The roles pharmacists can play in resolving the problem of noncompliance are varied. Home visits by pharmacists have been suggested by some (Schneider & Barber, 1996). A more complete integration into the traditional primary health care team has been proposed elsewhere (Bond et al., 1995). Pegrum (1995) has proposed the delivery of "seamless care" by and between community and hospital pharmacists through enhanced communication and interaction, and sharing of information between the two practice sites. Consumers themselves are expecting more from pharmacists as well (Morrow, Hargie, & Woodman, 1993). More and more patients expect advice, explanation, and information to enhance patient understanding.

Where does the pharmacist enter the compliance milieu? The potential for pharmacists to impact upon medication noncompliance is both enormous and rewarding. The pharmacist is the focal professional with regard to patient medication consumption. All points lead to the pharmacist, so to speak. The convergence of the marketing, prescribing, obtaining, and provision of product centers around the pharmacist. This convergence applies in all health care settings, whether ambulatory or institutional. Physicians who dispense medications to patients exclude pharmacists from the dispensing process. But in the vast majority of dispensing situations, pharmacists are the medication dispensers, and the potential for impact by the pharmacist may be the untapped answer for many of the problems of medication noncompliance. The provision of pharmaceutical care entails the dispensing of knowledge as well. Proper use of a drug may not occur without proper delivery of drug knowledge to the patient.

There is no professional in a better position to first detect, as well as inform others of, the noncompliant patient. Often, the pharmacist has a special relationship with both physician and patient. Due to this relationship, the pharmacist may "bridge the gap" between the wishes of the physician and the special problems and/or concerns of the patient. Considering the role of the pharmacist in the provision of pharmaceuticals to patients, the pharmacist also may be the professional to key upon with regard to strategic, mechanical, or behavioral attempts to impact upon the noncompliant patient.

NONCOMPLIANCE AS AN ALTERNATIVE

Noncompliance may seem to some patients as a viable alternative to complying with drug therapy regimens, especially when a patient may have definite opposing viewpoints to those of a physician.

Weintraub (1976) referred to patients purposely not complying with medication regimens and stated that patients' reasons for not complying seem to be valid in some cases. Elsewhere, noncompliance with mood-altering drugs may be a response by patients asserting their independence from psychiatric treatment (Kaplan, 1997).

The late Ivan Illich (1976) perhaps stated it best when he suggested: "To take a drug, no matter which and for what reason—is a last chance to assert control over himself, to interfere on his own with his own body rather than let others interfere" (p. 70).

Estimation of Noncompliance Rates

Various authors have estimated, in passing, the rate of compliance to be between 30 and 80 percent (Haynes, McDonald, & Garg, 2002). Rates for estimated compliance can vary as much as the differences between the samples studied and the therapeutic focus of interest in the study designs. Investigators fifty years ago narrowed their investigation of noncompliance to specific diseases that are treated by very narrow ranges of drug therapies. In an early study of noncompliance conducted five years ago with penicillin regimens to treat streptococcal infections, 34.3 percent of a sample was found to have taken less than the prescribed course of therapy (Mohler, Wallin, & Dreyfuss, 1955). Whether the effort is general or specific with regard to estimating noncompliance, Blackwell (1973) pointed out that there is neither an archetypal drug defaulter nor a single, simple solution to the puzzle of noncompliance.

THE CONSEQUENCES OF NONCOMPLIANCE

One of the inherent assumptions in many of the studies of noncompliance is that benefits in treatment outcomes will follow good patient compliance. There has been a virtual dearth of studies relating patient outcomes to noncompliance. Various authors have commented on the lack of a positive, definitive linking of noncompliance to deleterious effects in patient outcomes.

Ramifications of Noncompliance

The ramifications of noncompliance may affect the prescription drugs available for use as well as the assessed utility of drugs currently in use. Goetghebeur and Shapiro (1996) question the validity of clinical trials for new therapies, especially when substantial variation in dosing intervals is expected. They suggest using a repeated outcome measures approach and also incorporating a diary approach for patients to record dosing information. Polock and Abdulla (1998) have questioned the accuracy of pill counts in the measurement of compliance in clinical drug trials. Pullar and Feeley (1990) suggest that confirmation of noncompliance may be assessed in clinical trials, but that compliance is harder to quantify.

Noncompliance and Emergency Room Visits and Hospitalization

In a study examining the revolving door admission–readmission phenomenon in a sample of chronically ill mental patients, alcohol and drug problems and noncompliance were identified as major factors related to mental facility readmissions (1995). Prince et al. (1992) have chronicled drug-related emergency room visits and hospitalizations in relation to noncompliance. A total of 2 percent of HMO emergency room visits were due to medication misadventures (Schneitman-McIntire, Farnen, Gordon, Chan, & Toy, 1996). In this study, underuse was the most common problem identified for adolescent patients and overuse the most common problem of elderly patients. In another analysis of emergency room admissions, 58 percent of 565 visits were due to patient noncompliance (Dennehy, Kishi, & Louie, 1996). The reality is that we barely recognize the significant influence of noncompliance on emergency room and hospital admission and readmission rates.

FACTORS AFFECTING COMPLIANCE

Despite the compilation of factors (illness related and/or patient specific), noncompliance still is a pervasive problem in many patients (Hayes & Lucas, 1999). Drug compliance is, therefore, an individual-specific response by patients that is variable and often unable to be predicted in any number of differing patients and/or diseases. Over 250 separate and distinct factors have been found to be related to compliance (Haynes, Taylor, & Sackett, 1979). The factors to be discussed in this section make up a portion, but not the total, of these over 250 factors.

Haynes (1979) after a review of compliance studies assessed various factors with respect to influencing compliance either positively or negatively. The factors were separated into categories related to the disease, referral process, the clinic, and the treatment. The factors and their effect upon compliance are presented here (in adapted form):

Factors in compliance	Effect on compliance
The disease	
mental illness, schizophrenia,	
paranoia, personality disorders	Negative
Symptoms present	Negative
Disability	Positive
Referral process	
time from referral to appointment	Negative
(e.g., long)	
The clinic	
waiting time (e.g., long)	Negative
individual appointment time	Positive
patient making own appointments	Positive
as opposed to physician making	
appointment	
The treatment	
parenteral (refers to injections,	Positive
either intravenous, intramuscular,	
or subcutaneous)	
duration (long)	Negative
number of medications	Negative
treatment prescribed	Negative
cost (increased)	Negative
safety containers (lock top,	Negative
child-resistant containers)	
erring or errant pharmacist	Negative
(e.g., making mistakes)	

Individual studies that have included factors shown to affect compliance will now be presented.

Satisfaction with care. Physician communication style and patient satisfaction with care are both positively correlated with higher rates of patient compliance (Bultman & Svarstad, 2000). The more the care provided in a patient-centered approach, the greater the patient satisfaction and likelihood of compliance with recommendations (Stevenson, Barry, Britten, Barber, & Bradley, 2000).

Age. The age of a patient has been shown to positively affect, negatively affect, or to have no effect upon compliance. The vast majority of studies have shown no significant correlation between age and compliance (Haynes et al., 1979). It is fruitless to examine compliance and age and assume that there is a causal link between these constructs.

Gender. Gender has not been shown to be a reliable predictor of compliance. The ratio of studies showing no relationship to those with a positive relationship regarding gender and compliance is over 2 to 1 (Haynes et al., 1979). It is discriminatory to assume males or females are more or less compliant than one another. In one study, women have been shown to suffer death from myocardial infarctions if noncompliant with medications (Gallagher, Viscoli, & Horwitz, 1993). Compliance is a major problem for all, regardless of gender.

Cost. Patient compliance has been shown to be negatively affected by the cost of prescription drugs (Andrade, 1998). As coverage for prescription drug coverage in insurance plans diminishes, compliance can be expected to diminish as well. Compliance diminishes with economic stress regardless of whether the condition is reflux disorder (Bloom, 1995), respiratory infections (Kuti, 2002; Van Barlingen, 1998), depressive disorders (Revicki, 1995), or general infectious disease treatments (Verghese, 1991).

Knowledge of the disease. Knowledge of a particular disease (causation, prognosis, cure possibility) has been shown to be positively related to compliance with cardiovascular disease, and specific lipid disorders (McCann, Bovbjerg, Brief, & Turner, 1995; McCann et al., 1996; McCann, Retzlaff, Walden, & Knopp, 1998).

Work disruption. Work disruption, as measured by the effort required to seek care and wait for services while taking time off from work, has been shown to be negatively related to compliance (Nutt, 2000). Many patients are paid on an hourly basis and not reimbursed or excused for time away from work to visit the clinic.

Income. Income has been shown to have a direct relationship with patient compliance. There are inherent problems in generalizing from these studies to other study populations. Often, there has not been enough of a range in income in the groups studied to allow for a definite link to be established between income and compliance. For example, if the patient compliance in a population studied is low, and the income range of the group is narrow (as is the case in many compliance studies), a low income will automatically be correlated with poor patient compliance due to the economic status of the study population and the study design of the experiment. A similar spurious result could occur if both the range of incomes and reported compliance were high. Generalization from these samples to a broader population would be incorrect.

Continuity of the physician–patient relationship. The presence of a continuous physician–patient relationship has been shown to have a positive influence on patient compliance (Stevenson et al., 2000).

Medication errors. Medication errors have a devastating effect upon patients, families, and, certainly, compliance. Medication errors increase emergency room visits and affect patients upon dismissal (Naylor, 1996). Data are difficult to qualify on this important compliance impediment (Garrard, 2001). Confusion and errors only enhance drug-taking problems of patients (Dennehy, Kishi, & Louie, 1996).

DOSING

It has been shown that noncompliance can result when prescribers change the dosage of previously prescribed therapies, but do not notify pharmacists of the adjusted dosage (Reid et al., 2006). If patients are not adequately informed by the physician of such changes, they would certainly be in a position to be noncompliant through no fault of their own.

Simple, well-designed dosage schedules are necessary to avoid tolerance, rebound phenomenon, and to improve compliance with oral nitrates to treat angina pectoris (Held & Olsson, 1995). Once-a-day dosing offers advantages with improved compliance; however, more dose-free days may also be a result of once-daily dosage forms (Waeber et al., 1994). One has to balance and decide whether partial compliance with multiple interval dosing is more advantageous than missing an entire day of therapy when a day's dose is entirely omitted (Eisen, Miller, Woodward, Spitznagel, & Przybeck, 1990; Garrett, 1996). There may be other advantages to once-daily therapies. In a study of arthritis patients, O'Connor et al. (O'Connor et al., 1993) found that compliance increased with once-daily regimen of ibuprofen. Patient symptoms also improved, even though the total daily dose of ibuprofen was reduced. Adverse effects also decreased with the long-acting ibuprofen formulation. Studies have found that patients develop routines and backup strategies to cope with the complexity of regimens, and to know under what circumstances they may be more prone to negative and noncompliant behaviors (Reid et al., 2006).

DEVICES TO AID PATIENT COMPLIANCE

Many devices have been used to try and improve patient compliance. These range from prescriber order entry by physicians (Segarra, DeStefano, & Davis, 1991) with the goal of decreasing prescription processing time and increasing the opportunities for pharmacists to work with patients. Computer-generated reminder charts for patients (Forcinio, 1993) and various caps and counter devices have also been tried.

Technology alone will not solve the vexing problem of noncompliance; in fact in some cases it may diminish compliance. In a study examining the combination of two inhaled asthma preparations in one inhaler (budesonide plus terbutaline sulphate) as a tool to increase compliance, the results were just the opposite (Bosley, Parry, & Cochrane, 1994). Only 15 percent of patients were compliant more than 80 percent of the time. The use of a tablet splitter to enable economic savings by dividing a higher-dose tablet into two smaller doses was found to discourage patients from complying because of confusion (Carr-Lopez, Mallett, & Morse, 1995). The use of a notched, clicking cap for prescription medications has been shown to increase compliance (Perri, Martin, & Pritchard, 1995). Caps imbedded with electronic devices that can then download information to track compliance have been used as compliance-detecting and recording tools (Cramer, 1995; Urquhart, 1993). Other electronic devices can measure removal compliance from blister-packaged doses (Wingender & Kuppers, 1993). Blister packaging and compliance packaging have been used to enhance compliance (Tiano, 1994). Unit-of-use blister packaging has been advocated for use in the United States. (Beagley, 1996). Blister packaging and unit-of-use materials are extensively used for prescription medications elsewhere in the world (Forcinio, 1993). However, unit-of-use packaging is not without controversy; it has in fact been criticized for lack of standardization in products by manufacturers, which can confuse patients (Rigby, 2002).

COMMUNICATION

Regardless of form, communication must be seen as the key component for increasing compliance. DiMatteo, Reiter, and Gambone (1994) have suggested the use of communication with patients to engender informed choices that in turn lead to enhanced communication. Lambert and Lee (1994) have noted that both content and design are crucial to success. Labeling techniques influence as well (Morrell, Park, & Poon, 1990). Roter (1995) promoted the use of a collaborative process when compliance difficulties arise.

MANUFACTURERS

Many manufacturers are attempting and succeeding in developing a personal relationship with patients. Increased name recognition, brand loyalty, establishing communication conduits, therapeutic switches, and potentials for increased product usage are but a few of the reasons for doing so. Pharmacists' responses to such manufacturer outreach programs vary. Smith and Basara (1996) in a national study found that most pharmacists believed that pharmacists should not be compensated for switching patients' therapies. An interesting finding was that respondents did not feel that patient compliance was a major problem. Elsewhere, Basara and Smith (1995) have noted that most pharmacists in the study felt that although the manufacturers' programs did benefit and improve compliance, the manufacturer should not be involved in patient education and compliance monitoring. They conclude that pharmacist–manufacturer relations may improve by incorporating pharmacists into the programs.

SUMMARY

Both self-medication and patient compliance behaviors are exceedingly complex. McDonald, Garg, and Haynes (2002) point out that patient interventions to impact compliance are complex, labor intensive, and not particularly effective. McDonald et al. (2002) further suggest that more convenient care, reminders, self-monitoring by patients, reinforcement, family therapy, and additional attention may need to be in play for compliance improvement to occur. Meredith (1998) notes that a focus on the individual, rather than a general approach, is more likely to be successful. Haynes and colleagues (2002) call for better approaches that are more efficient and more effective in enhancing compliance .

REFERENCES

Andrade, S. (1998). Compliance in the real world. *Value Health, 1*(3): 171-173.
Barry, K. (1993). Patient self-medication: An innovative approach to medication teaching. *J Nurs Care Qual, 8*: 75-82.
Basara, L. R., & Smith, M. C. (1995). Pharmacist perspectives on patient programs. *Pharm Exec, 15*(November): 83-86.
Beagley, K. G. (1996). Will unit-of-use take off? *Pharm & Med Pack News, 4*(6): 20-21, 24, 28.
Bero, L., & Blackwell, B. (1973). Patient compliance. *N Engl J Med, 289*: 249-252.
Bloom, B. S. (1995). Cost and quality effects of treating erosive esophagitis: Re-evaluation. *PharmacoEconomics, 8*(August): 139-146.
Bond, C. M., Sinclair, H. K., Taylor, R. J., Duffus, P., Reid, J., & Williams, A. (1995). Pharmacists: Resource for general practice? *Int J Pharm Pract, 3* (March): 85-90.
Bosley, C. M., Parry, D. T., & Cochrane, G. M. (1994). Patient compliance with inhaled medication: Does combining beta-agonists with corticosteroids improve compliance? *Eur Respir J, 7*(3): 504-509.
Bruzek, R. (1994). Community pharmacist: Delivering quality care and lower costs. *AAPPOJ, 4*(November-December): 32, 35-36.
Bultman, D. C., & Svarstad, B. L. (2000). Effects of physician communication style on client medication beliefs and adherence with antidepressant treatment. *Soc Sci Med, 40*: 173-185.

Carr-Lopez, S. M., Mallett, M. S., & Morse, T. (1995). Tablet splitter: Barrier to compliance or cost-saving instrument? *Am J Health Syst Pharm, 52*(December 1): 2707-2708.

Catford, J. (1995). Health promotion in the marketplace: Constraints and opportunities. *Health Prom Int, 10*(1): 41-50.

Cramer, J. A. (1995). Microelectronic systems for monitoring and enhancing patient compliance with medication regimens. *Drugs, 49*(March): 321-327.

Dean, K. (1986). Lay care in illness. *Soc Sci Med, 22*(2): 275-284.

Dennehy, C. E., Kishi, D. T., & Louie, C. (1996). Drug-related illness in emergency department patients. *Am J Health Syst Pharm, 53*(12): 1422-1426.

DiMatteo, M. R., Reiter, R. C., & Gambone, J. C. (1994). Enhancing medication adherence through communication and informed collaborative choice. *Health Communication, 5*: 253-266.

Eisen, S. A., Miller, D. K., Woodward, R. S., Spitznagel, E., & Przybeck, T. R. (1990). The effect of prescribed daily dose frequency on patient medication compliance. *Arch of Int Med, 150*: 1881-1884.

Elliott, W. J. (1994). Compliance strategies. *Curr Opin Nephrol Hypertens, 3*(3): 271-278.

Family Core Component of the 1997-2004 National Health Interview Surveys, U.S. Centers for Disease Control, Atlanta, GA. http://www.cdc.gov/nchs/data/nhis/earlyrelease/200506_01.pdf. Accessed July 25, 2005.

Fawcett, J. (1995). Compliance: Definitions and key issues. *J Clin Psychiatry, 56*(1): 4-8.

Forcinio H. (1993). Packaging solutions that help patient compliance. *Pharm Technol, 17*(March): 44, 46, 48, 50.

Gallagher, E. J., Viscoli, C. M., & Horwitz, R. (1993). The relationship of treatment adherence to the risk of death after myocardial infraction in women. *JAMA, 270*: 742-744.

Gannon, K. (1991). Switched drugs lend vitality to surging OTC market. *Drug Topics, 135*(May 20): 32, 36.

Garrard, J. (2001). Management and prevention of medication errors in managed care organizations. *Prevent Med Manag Care, 2*(2): 61-73.

Garrett, S. S. (1996). Deciding between once- and twice-daily dosing. *Am J Health Syst Pharm, 53*(April 1): 730-731. .

Goetghebeur, E. J. T., & Shapiro, S. (1996). Analyzing non-compliance in clinical trials: Ethical imperative or mission impossible. *Stat Med, 15*: 2813-2826.

Hayes, G., & Lucas, B. (1999). Tools for improving compliance. *Pat Care, 33*(15): 15-16.

Haynes, R. B. (1979). Determinants of compliance: The disease and mechanics of treatment. In Haynes, R. B., Taylor, D. W., Sackett, D. L., (Eds.), *Compliance in health care* (pp. 49-62). Baltimore: Johns Hopkins University Press.

Haynes, R. B., McDonald, H. P., & Garg, A. X. (2002). Helping patients follow prescribed treatment. *JAMA, 288*(22): 2880-2883.

Haynes, R. B., Taylor, D. W., & Sackett, D. L., (Eds.) (1979). *Compliance in health care*. Baltimore: Johns Hopkins University Press.

Held, P., & Olsson, G. (1995). The rationale for nitrates in angina pectoris. *Can J Cardiol, 11* (Supplement B): 11B-13B.

Illich, I. (1976). *Medical nemesis.* New York: Bantam Books.

Isaac, L. M., & Tamblyn, R. M. (1993). Compliance and cognitive function: A methodological approach to measuring unintentional errors in medication compliance in the elderly. *Gerontologist, 33*: 772-781.

Janoff, B. (1999). Making the switch. *Prog Groc, 78*(5): 135-136.

Kaplan, E. M. (1997). Antidepressant noncompliance as a factor in the discontinuation syndrome. *J Clin Psych, 58*(7): 31-36.

Kelly, J. M. (1994). Implementing a patient self-medication program. *Rehabil Nurs, 19*(2): 87-90.

Kjellgren, K. I., Ahlner, J., & Saljo, R. (1995). Taking hypertensive medication— controlling or co-operating with patients? *Int J Cardiol, 47*(3): 257-268.

Kogan. M. D., Pappas, G., Yu, S. M., & Kotelchuck, M. (1994). Over-the-counter medication use among U.S. preschool-age children. *JAMA, 272*: 1025-1030.

Kuti, J. L. (2002). Cost-effective approaches to the treatment of community-acquired pneumonia in the era of resistance. *PharmacoEcon, 20*(8): 513-528.

Lambert, B. L., & Lee, J. Y. (1994). Patient perceptions of pharmacy students' hypertension compliance gaining messages: Effects of message design logic and content themes. *Health Comm, 6*(4): 311-326.

McCann, B.S. Bovbjerg, V.E., Brief, D. J., & Turner, W. C. (1995). Relationship of self-efficacy to cholesterol lowering and dietary change in hyperlipidemia. *Ann Behav Med, 17*(3): 221-226.

McCann, B. S., Bovbjerg, V. E., Curry, S. J., Retzlaff, B. M, Walden, C. E., & Knopp R. H (1996). Predicting participation in a dietary intervention to lower cholesterol among individuals with hyperlipidemia. *Health Psych,* (1): 61-64.

McCann, B. S., Retzlaff, B. M., Walden, C. E., & Knopp, R. H. (1998). Dietary intervention for coronary heart disease. In Shumaker, Sally A. Schron, Eleanor B. et al. (Eds.), *The handbook of health behavioral change* (pp. 191-215). New York: Springer Publishing Co.

McDonald, H. P., Garg, A. X., & Haynes, R. B. (2002). Interventions to enhance patient adherence to medication prescriptions. *JAMA, 288*(22): 2868-2879.

Meredith, P. A. (1998). Enhancing patients' compliance. *BMJ, 316*: 393-394.

Miller, J. L. (2001). A perfect storm: The confluence of forces affecting health care coverage. Washington, DC: National Coalition on Health Care.

Mohler D. N., Wallin, D. G., & Dreyfus, E. G. (1955). Studies in the home treatment of streptococcal disease, failure of patients to take penicillin by mouth as prescribed. *N Engl J Med, 252*: 1116-1118.

Morrell, R. W., Park, D. C., & Poon, L. W. (1990). Effects of labeling techniques on memory and comprehension of prescription information in young and old adults. *J Geron, 45*: 166-172.

Morrow, N., Hargie, O., & Woodman, C. (1993). Consumer perceptions of and attitudes to the advice-giving role of community pharmacists. *Pharm J, 251*(July 3): 25-27.

Naylor, D. M. (1996). Assessing the need for a domiciliary pharmaceutical service for elderly patients using a coding system to record and quantify data. *Pharm J, 258*(April 5): 479-484.

Nutt, D. (2000). Treatment of depression and concomitant anxiety. *European Neuropsychopharmacology, 10*(l4): S433-S437.

O' Connor, T. P., Anderson, A. M., Lennox, B., & Muldoon, C. (1993). Novel sustained-release formulation of ibuprofen provides effective once-daily therapy in the treatment of rheumatoid arthritis and osteoarthritis. *Br J Clin Pract, 47*(1): 10-13.

Ory, M. G., DeFriese, G. H., & Duncker, A. P. (1998). Introduction. In Ory, M. G. & DeFriese, G. H. (Eds.), *Self-care in later life* (pp. xv-xxvi). New York: Springer Publishing Company.

Pegrum S. (1995). Seamless care: Need for communication between hospital and community pharmacists. *Pharm J, 254*(April 1): 445-446.

Perri, M., Martin, B. C., & Pritchard, F. L. (1995). Improving medication compliance: Practical intervention. *J Pharm Technol,* 11(July-August): 167-172.

Polock, S., & Abdulla, M. (1998). The hope and hazards of using compliance data in randomized controlled trials. *Statistics in Medicine, 17*: 303-317.

Prince, B. S., Goetz, C. M., Rihn, T. L., & Olsky, M. (1992). Drug-related emergency department visits and hospital admissions. *A J Hosp Pharm, 49*: 1696-1700.

Pullar T., & Feeley, M. P. (1990). Reporting compliance in clinical trials. *Lancet, 336*: 1253-1254.

Reid, M., Clark, A. et al. (2006). Patients strategies for managing medication for chronic heart failure. *Int J Cardiol, 109*(1): 66-73.

Revicki, D. A. (1995). Modeling the cost effectiveness of antidepressant treatment in primary care. *PharmacoEconomics, 8*(December): 524-540.

Rigby, M. (2002). Pharmaceutical packaging can induce confusion. *BMJ, 324*: 679.

Roter, D. (1995). Advancing the physician's contribution to enhancing compliance. *J Pharmacoepidem, 3*(2): 37-48.

Sbarbaro, J. A., & Steiner, J. F. (1991). Noncompliance with medications: Vintage wine in new (pill) bottles. *Ann Allerg, 66*: 273-275.

Schneider, J., & Barber, N. (1996). Provision of a domiciliary service by community pharmacists. *Int J Pharm Pract, 4*(March): 19-24.

Schneitman-McIntire, O., Farnen, T. A., Gordon, N., Chan, J., & Toy, W. A. (1996). Medication misadventures resulting in emergency department visits at an HMO medical center. *Am J Health Syst Pharm, 53*(June 15): 1416-1422.

Segarra, J., DeStefano, J. J., & Davis, R. H. (1991). Streamlining outpatient prescription dispensing utilizing prescriber order entry. *ASHP Midyear Clinical Meeting, 26*(December): P-425D.

Smith, M., & Basara, L. (1996). Pharmacists' opinions about manufacturers' outreach programs. *J Am Pharm Assn, NS36*(August): 497-502.

Smith, M. B., & Feldman, W. (1993). Over-the-counter cold medication: Critical review of clinical trials between 1950 and 1991. *JAMA, 269*: 2258-2263.

Stevenson, F. A., Barry, C. A., Britten, N., Barber, N., & Bradley, C. P. (2000). Doctor-patient communication about drugs: The evidence for shared decision making. *Soc Sci Med, 50*: 829-840.

Stoller, E. P., Forster, L. E., & Portugal, P. (1993). Self-care response to symptoms by older people: A health diary study of illness behavior. *Med Care, 31*(1): 24-42.

Tiano, F. J. (1994). Compliant packaging. *Clin Res Regul Aff, 11*(1): 39-46.

Urquhart, J. (1993). When outpatient drug treatment fails: Identifying noncompliers as a cost-containment tool. *Med Interface, 6*(April): 65-67, 71-73.

Van Barlingen, H. J. (1998). Model to evaluate the cost-effectiveness of different antibiotics in the management of acute bacterial exacerbations of chronic bronchitis in Germany. *J Med Econ, 1*: 201-218.

Verghese, A. (1991). Use of oral antibiotics in daily clinical practice. *Drugs, 42*(4): 1-5.

Waeber, B., Erne, P., Saxenhofer, H. et al. (1994). Use of drugs with more than a twenty-four hour duration of action. *J Hypertension Supplement, 12*(8): S67-71.

Weiland J. (1996). Are patients at risk in their attempts to self medicate with OTC products? *MD Pharm, 72*(March-April): 26-28.

Weinstein, A. G. (1995). Clinical management strategies to maintain drug compliance in asthmatic children. *Ann Allergy Asthma Immunol, 74*: 304-310.

Weintraub, M. (1976). Intelligent noncompliance and capricious compliance. In Lasagna, L., (Ed.), *Patient compliance.* Mt. Kisco, NY: Futura Publishing Company.

Wingender, W., & Kuppers, J. (1993). Bayer compliance device. *Drug Inf J, 27*(4): 1103-1106.

Chapter 3

Drug Therapies Leading to Noncompliant Activity

Jayashri Sankaranarayanan

INTRODUCTION

The purpose of this chapter is to provide a brief introduction to compliance, often referred to as adherence, and an overview of the drug therapies that lead to patient noncompliance. For this purpose, based on literature, information on (1) the structure and demands of various therapies, (2) the common themes of patient attributes, and (3) health professional attributes that affect compliance are presented and discussed.

The best treatment can be rendered ineffective by poor adherence. Treatment effectiveness leading to optimal outcomes in population health is determined jointly by the efficacy of the treatment and the extent of adherence to the treatment. Despite the availability of efficacious interventions, treatment nonadherence is the single most important modifiable factor that compromises treatment outcome, cost, and effectiveness across therapeutic areas (WHO, 2003).

Worldwide, poor adherence is well recognized but inadequately addressed and understudied as a major public health cause for the gap

The author of this chapter would like to thank Dr. Holly L. Mason, associate dean for academic programs and professor of pharmacy administration at the College of Pharmacy, Nursing and Health Sciences, Purdue University, West Lafayette, Indiana, for review and comments on this chapter.

between optimal and usual care in many therapeutic areas. It is often referred to as the nation's other drug problem (Bender & Rand, 2004; Elliott, Barber, & Horne, 2005; Wahl et al., 2005; WHO, 2003). Specifically, patients' failure to adhere to health professionals' recommendations and medication nonadherence are reported to cost as much as $300 billion to the healthcare systems in the United States (Bender & Rand, 2004). Poor adherence to recognized standards of care is the principal cause of development of complications of medical conditions, wastage of resources, preventable morbidity and mortality, loss of health care dollars and productivity, all of which are associated with individual, societal, and economic costs (Oldridge, 2001; WHO, 2003).

Empirical studies have consistently found that levels of compliance or adherence are often far from optimal (WHO, 2003). Health outcomes between high and low adherence is reported to be 26 percent, and the adherence–outcome relationship varies with the regimens, measurements, and diseases studied (DiMatteo, Giordani, Lepper, & Groghan, 2002). Health care costs vastly differ between patients with high and low adherence, with a clear relationship seen between increased medication adherence, improved health outcomes, and lower health care costs (Aday, Begley, Lairson, & Balkrishnan, 2004; Balkrishnan et al., 2003).

Recently, Sokol and colleagues (2005) showed that in four chronic conditions (hypertension, health failure, diabetes, and hypercholesterolemia) higher medication costs driven by improved adherence with guidelines-based therapy and higher medication adherence were found to reduce disease-related costs (e.g., lower hospitalization rates and costs). These savings produced a net economic return. This establishes the role of medication utilization and adherence in the effective management of chronic diseases with lower overall avoidable health care utilization and morbidity. Similarly, poor (~50 percent) adherence to inhaled corticosteroids among adult asthmatics was correlated with several poor asthma-related outcomes including a majority of asthma-related hospitalizations (Williams et al., 2004). Medication underuse (a gap from one to more than thirty days of medications) in schizophrenic outpatients prescribed antipsychotics was associated with greater risk of hospitalization among all other risk factors (Weiden, Kozma, Grogg, & Locklear, 2004). Hence, for its effects on health and provider services, informal caregivers, employers, and society, research on medication adherence is considered the next major therapeutic advancement (Elliott, Barber, & Horne, 2005).

MEDICATION ADHERENCE OR COMPLIANCE: DEFINITIONS, ESTIMATES, MEASUREMENT, AND INTERVENTIONS

Patient compliance presents difficult issues on both conceptual and methodological levels in many aspects.

Definitions

A recent WHO report (2003) used the following comprehensive definition of adherence to long-term therapy: "Adherence is the extent to which a person's behavior—taking medication, following a diet, and/or executing lifestyle changes, corresponds with agreed recommendations from a health care provider" (Haynes, 1979; *Merriam-Webster,* 2005; Rand, 1993; Sackett & Haynes, 1976; WHO, 2003). Medication adherence has also been referred to as the level of participation achieved in a medication regimen once a patient has agreed to the regimen (Mihalko et al., 2004). To date, the terms compliance and adherence, used interchangeably, imply patient behavior being congruent with health care providers' recommendations (Elliott, Barner, & Horne, 2005). However, these broad definitions underestimate the complexity of the issue.

Estimates

Estimates of noncompliance or nonadherence with prescribed therapeutic regimens typically range from 15 to 93 percent (Balkrishnan, 2005; Singh et al., 1996). An average estimated rate of 25 to 50 percent of patients for whom drugs are prescribed fail to receive full benefit due to inadequate adherence (Fincham, 1995; Kravitz & Melnikow, 2004; Rogers & Bullman, 1995; Roter et al., 1998). About half of all patients with chronic diseases have been known to stop refilling prescriptions within a year (Wahl et al., 2005). People who are prescribed self-administered medications typically take less than half the prescribed doses (Haynes, McDonald, Garg, & Montague, 2002). According to one estimate almost one-third of patients who received prescriptions were using them in a manner that posed a serious threat to their health (Boyd, Covington, Stanaszek, & Coussons, 1974).

Measurement and Interventions

Nonadherence will always exist and the method of assessment matters (DiMatteo, 2004). There is no "gold" standard for measuring adherence behavior, since there is no single, sufficiently reliable, and accurate method. The most commonly used methods are traditional subjective measures (patient self-report, patient interviews, using health care providers' or caregiver judgment as proxy reports), and objective measures (physical measures such as pill counts, reviewing prescription refill patterns, electronic measurement devices, clinical outcome measures, and measurement of blood or urine concentrations of the drug). Both methods may overestimate adherence and may not be accurate (Balkrishnan, 2005; Elliott, Barber, & Horne, 2005; MacLaughlin et al., 2005; WHO, 2003). Further, objective adherence measurements may be confounded by treatment type (since medication adherence, measured objectively, tends to run higher than lifestyle adherence) (DiMatteo, 2004; Kravitz & Melnikow, 2004).

The accuracy of self-reported adherence is compromised by recall, and self-presentational/social desirability biases. Recall bias occurs when respondents cannot remember precise details of adherence or do not accurately recall their levels of adherence over a period of time. Self-presentational or social desirability bias occurs when patients intentionally exaggerate their level of adherence in an attempt to avoid being perceived negatively. The expense of technological devices (like electronic medication event monitoring system [MEMS], which record the time and date when a medication container is opened) to improve adherence limits their widespread use. Pharmacy databases are used to study when prescriptions are initially filled, refilled over time, and prematurely discontinued. They measure when the medicine was obtained but do not measure its actual use. Also, such information can be incomplete because patients may use more than one pharmacy or data may not be routinely captured. Several of the measurement strategies are costly (e.g., MEMS) or depend on information technology (e.g., pharmacy databases) that is unavailable in many countries.

In summary, measurement of adherence provides useful information that outcome-monitoring alone cannot provide, but it remains only an estimate of a patient's actual behavior. A multi-method approach that combines feasible self-reporting and reasonable objective measures is the current recommendation for measurement of adherence behavior (Balkrishnan, 2005; Elliott, Barber & Horne, 2005; MacLaughlin et al., 2005; WHO, 2003). Independent of the measurement technique used, thresholds defining "good" and "bad" adherence in practice might not really exist because the dose-response phenomenon is a continuum function. Although dose-response curves are difficult to construct for real-life situations, where dosage, timing, and other variables might be different from those tested in clinical trials, they are needed if sound policy decisions are to be made when defining operational adherence thresholds for different therapies (WHO, 2003).

Interventions

Compared to any improvement in specific medical treatments, increasing the effectiveness of adherence interventions is expected to have a far greater impact on the health of the population. Hence, there is growing interest in developing innovative patient adherence interventions to assist patients in the following recommendations for prescribed medications (Haynes, McDonald, Garg, & Montague, 2002; McDonald, Garg, & Haynes, 2002). Adherence interventions need to be not only effective but also cost effective. So they should be informed by theory, based on causes for nonadherence, and should be targeted at key patient groups (Elliott, Barber, & Horne, 2005). Adherence interventions have many designs: combinations of more convenient care, information, counseling, reminders, self-monitoring, telling patients about adverse effects of treatment, reinforcement, family therapy, and other forms of additional supervision or attention by a health care provider (physician, nurse, pharmacist, or other). Their drawbacks include no theoretical basis; narrow and limited interventions; methodologies and operational definitions of adherence as varied as the diseases, regimens, and patients; measurement and context differences producing wide variations in adherence estimates, correlates, and outcomes; and use of intensive multicomponent interventions unlikely to be transferable to normal care. There were also difficulties in definitions of interventions where effects were due only to changes in medication adherence and in problematic associations of adherence to improved outcomes (Elliott, Barber, & Horne, 2005; DiMatteo, Lepper, & Croghan, 2000; DiMatteo et al., 2002; Roter et al., 1998; Vik, Maxwell, & Hogan, 2004; Trostel, 1997). Compliance intervention studies need to address the broader spectrum of patient outcomes, valued by health services researchers, such as satisfaction, physician communication behavior to patient outcomes, patient empowerment, comprehension and understanding, as well as markers of clinical significance including quality of life, functional status, and enhancement of emotional health and well-being (Roter et al., 1998) across multiple conditions. Thus, the full benefits of medications would remain unrealized at currently achievable levels of adherence (Haynes, McDonald, Garg, & Montague, 2002; McDonald, Garg, & Haynes, 2002). For this purpose it is important to understand the theoretical aspects of medication adherence, which are now discussed.

THEORETICAL ASPECTS

The epidemiological shift in disease burden from acute to chronic diseases over the past fifty years has led to a shift from the inadequate acute care models of health service delivery to chronic care models to address the health needs of the population. Behavioral science offers useful theories, models, and strategies that support best-practice approaches to delivering treatment and help to explain behavioral change in nonadherence. The effectiveness of adherence interventions based on behavioral principles has been demonstrated in many therapeutic areas. Examples include hypertension, headache, Acquired Immunodeficiency Syndrome (AIDS), cancer, heart transplantation, chronic asthma, diabetes, high cholesterol, obesity, sun-protection, and smoking cessation behaviors.

Decades of behavioral research and practice have yielded proven strategies for changing people's behavior in diverse medical conditions, which can also be effective in changing the behavior of health care providers and health care systems (WHO, 2003). Leventhal and Cameron (1994) outlined five general theoretical perspectives on adherence: (1) the dominant biomedical perspective, which assumes that patients are more or less passive followers of their doctor's orders, after a diagnosis and prescribed therapy; (2) behavioral perspective, which emphasizes the importance of positive and negative reinforcement as a mechanism for influencing adherence behavior; (3) communication perspective, which emerged in the 1970s, encouraged health care providers to improve their skills in communicating with their patients; (4) cognitive perspective; emphasizing cognitive variables and processes applied to adherence behavior. Common model components involve patients' cognitive and social processes (e.g., beliefs, norms), and patients' resources (e.g., financial, psychological, and social support). These approaches have directed attention to the ways in which patients conceptualize health threats and appraise factors that may be barriers to, or facilitate, adherence but do not always address behavioral coping skills; and (5) self-regulatory perspective attempts to integrate environmental variables and the cognitive responses of individuals to health threats into the self-regulatory model. Other theoretical models used to explain intentional nonadherence are the necessity-concerns framework and the application of human error that encompasses causes of unintentional and intentional nonadherence such as cost, patient–professional relationships, levels of knowledge, and drug acceptability (Barber, 2002; Elliott, Barber, & Horne, 2005).

The medication use process by patients is a complex process in the United States. From the point of seeking medical care for their symptoms, patients have to encounter various predisposing, enabling, and need factors that impact their behavioral utilization of medical care services, which includes treatment with medications. A comprehensive framework for analyses originated from Andersen and Newman, who proposed the model of behavioral utilization consisting of the three (predisposing, enabling, and need) factors, which interact in various ways and produce a continuum of utilization for various medical care services (Andersen & Newman, 1973). Andersen and Newman were among the first to consider contextual variables like the health system variables in their framework of behavioral health care utilization. Authors and researchers have adapted this framework to their research while some others are identifying variables affecting adherence, and this is an ongoing process. Some of the variables identified can represent more than one kind of factor. For example, the delivery system variables like third-party coverage, pharmacy services, medical practices, institutionalization, and marketing practices can be predisposing and enabling and/or need factor determinants of the medication use and adherence behavior (Smith, 1996). The empirical literature on adherence is large but not well understood, even with elegant conceptual frameworks (Bowen, Helmes, & Lease, 2001). However, a considerable amount of empirical and descriptive research has identified correlates and predictors of adherence and nonadherence and is used in the following discussion.

STRUCTURE AND DEMAND OF DRUG THERAPIES

The risk of poor adherence increases with the structure and demand of drug therapies. Adherence is a complex behavioral process determined by several interacting factors. These include aspects of the complexity and duration of treatment, characteristics of the illness, iatrogenic effects of treatment (both long duration and complex treatment [including behavioral modifications] inherent to chronic illnesses), costs of treatment, characteristics of health service provision, interaction between practitioner and patient, and sociodemographic variables, many of which may not be amenable to intervention. Several important variables that are behavioral are dynamic, and are, therefore, amenable to intervention (WHO, 2003).

The treatments that patients are asked to follow vary according to the nature of the demands they impose. They range from requiring relatively simple and familiar behaviors to more complex and novel ones. Some treatments involve one behavior, while others carry multiple behavioral requirements. Protocols also vary in terms of the length of time for which they must be followed. Patients may not adhere to many specific aspects of treatment, for example health-seeking behaviors (like appointment keeping); obtaining inoculations;

medication use (use of appropriate agents, correct dosing and timing, filling and refilling prescriptions, consistency of use, duration of use); and following protocols for changing behavior (examples include modifying diet, increasing physical activity, quitting smoking, self-monitoring of symptoms, safe food handling, dental hygiene, and safer injection practices). This means that the nature and meaning of adherence changes with specific treatment demands of a patient. Patients differ in their ability to meet those demands, and the resources available and the environmental contexts also differ. Reflecting on the process of efforts occurring over the course of an illness to meet the treatment-related behavioral demands imposed by that illness would contribute to defining adherence more explicitly according to the type of behavior, an acceptable frequency, consistency, intensity, and/or accuracy (WHO, 2003).

Collaborative efforts to improve adherence to treatments for chronic illness, recently promoted by the WHO, must include multiple components of the health care system (Bender & Rand, 2004; WHO, 2003). Adherence is a multidimensional phenomenon determined by the simultaneous interaction of many "dimensions or factors," of which patient-related is just one determinant. The common belief that patients are solely responsible for taking their treatment is misleading and most often reflects a misunderstanding of how other factors affect people's behavior and capacity to adhere to their treatment. In order to identify multiple components of adherence, it is important to continually understand the dimensions of adherence proposed by the WHO defined "health care team," which are condition-related factors, medication therapy related factors; and patient-related factors, social- and economic-related factors; and health system/health care team-related factors (WHO, 2003). To conserve space, the health system factors are included with health professional attributes, and social- and economic-related factors are included with the patient attributes in the discussion here (see and Figure 3.1). The key medical condition and medication therapy related factors, patients-related factors, and health professional attributes, and health system factors of adherence are presented here.

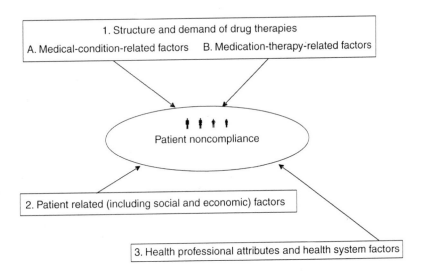

FIGURE 3.1. Factors related to adherence. *Source:* Adapted from World Health Organization (2005). *Adherence to long-term therapies-evidence for action* (2003). Available at: http://www.who.int/chronic_conditions/en/adherence_ report.pdf.

MEDICAL-CONDITION-RELATED FACTORS

The variation in adherence across medical conditions represents a tremendous challenge to population health efforts where success is determined primarily by adherence to long-term therapies (WHO, 2003). For example, in developed countries, such as the United States, only 51 percent of the patients treated for hypertension adhere to the prescribed treatment. Between 40 and 70 percent of patients with depression adhere to antidepressant therapies. In Australia, only 43 percent of the patients with asthma take their medication as prescribed all the time and only 28 percent use prescribed preventive medication. In the treatment of Human Immunodeficiency Virus infection (HIV) and AIDS, adherence to antiretroviral agents varies between 37 and 95 percent depending on the drug under study and patient population demographics. Adherence is reported to be around 66 percent for diabetes and sleep disorders (DiMatteo, 2004; WHO, 2003).

Based on the WHO (2003) report, DiMatteo's (2004) review, and literature reports, adherence for medical conditions is varied (see Table 3.1). These assessments may be overestimates and not generalizable to real-world settings, because they are drawn from multiple sources limited to the adherence context of physician–patient relationship based on medical recommendations. However, the reported adherence estimates ranged from 5 to 96 percent across various medical conditions and therapies and do highlight poor adherence even in the presence of medical recommendations (DiMatteo, 2004; Smith, 1996; WHO, 2003).

Even though the number of studies conducted in these areas may limit generalizability of findings, enhancement of compliance for some conditions is either more difficult or less efficacious in producing positive patient outcomes than for other conditions. Particularly, compliance interventions showed stronger benefits for patients with particular chronic conditions and were especially effective for diabetes; more moderately so for asthma, cancer, hypertension, and mental illness; and weaker for acute conditions such as otitis media and unspecified conditions (usually infections, for which antibiotics were prescribed). Similarly, premature discontinuation of statins can be substantial, because patients may be doubtful of the necessity of the treatment in asymptomatic hypercholesterolemia (Peterson & McGhan, 2005). There is no single intervention strategy, or package of strategies, that has been shown to be effective across all patients, conditions, and settings. Consequently, interventions that target adherence must be tailored to the particular illness-related demands experienced and a patient-specific approach should be modeled (DiMatteo, 2004; WHO, 2003).

In summary, condition-related factors (see Table 3.2) represent particular illness-related demands faced by the patient. Some strong determinants of adherence are those related to the severity of symptoms, level of disability (physical, psychological, social, and vocational), rate of progression and severity of the disease, and the availability of effective treatments. Their impact depends on how they influence patients' risk perception, the importance of following treatment, and the priority placed on adherence. Comorbidities, such as depression (in diabetes or HIV/AIDS), and drug and alcohol abuse are important modifiers of adherence behavior (WHO, 2003).

TABLE 3.1. Adherence rates in various medical conditions or for various therapies.

Medical conditions/therapies	Range of adherence rates (Reference) %
Immunosuppressant therapy in solid organ transplantation	5-70 [5]
Asthma	20-43 [1,2,3]
Anticoagulation	30-50 [4]
Seizures/brain disorders including epilepsy	30-96 [1,3]
HIV disease	37-95 [1,2]
Cardio vascular diseases(including adherence for hypertension and other cardiovascular disease)	40-80 [1,2,3]
Diabetes	40-76 [1,3]
Depression	40-70 [2]
Blood disorders (not leukemia)	46-96 [1]
Sleep disorders	54-76 [1,2]
Arthritis	55-89 [1,3]
End-stage renal disease	57-82 [1]
Pulmonary diseases	61-76 [1]
Eye disorders	62-82 [1]
Obstetric and gynecological disorders	64-84 [1]
Genitourinary and sexually transmitted diseases (STDs)	66-87 [1]
Skin disorders	67-86 [1]
Infectious disease	68-80 [1]
Ear, nose, throat, and mouth disorders	69-83 [1]
Gastrointestinal disorders	74-86 [1]
Cancer	76-84 [1]

Notes:
[1]DiMatteo, R. (2004). Variations in patients' adherence to medical recommendations: A quantitative review of 50 years of research. *Med Care*, 42: 200-209.
[2]World Health Organization (2005). *Adherence to long-term therapies-evidence for action* (2003). Available at: http://www.who.int/chronic_conditions/en/adherence_report.pdf.
[3]Smith, M. C. (1996). Predicting and detecting noncompliance. In Smith, M. C. & Werthei-mer, A. I., (Eds.), *Social and behavioral aspects of pharmaceutical care*. Binghamton, NY: The Haworth Press.
[4]Davis, N. J., Billett, H. H., Cohen, H. W., & Arnsten, J. H. (2005). Impact of adherence, knowledge, and quality of life on anticoagulation control. *Ann Pharmacother*, 39(4): 632-636.
[5]Chisholm, M. A., Lance, C. E., Williamson, G. M., & Mulloy, L. L. (2005). Development and validation of an immunosuppressant therapy adherence barrier instrument. *Nephrol Dial Transplant*, 20(1): 181-188.

TABLE 3.2. Medical-condition-related factors of adherence.

Asymptomatic disease (−)
Poor understanding of disease and treatment side effects (−)
Depression (−)
Psychiatric comorbidities (−)
Chronic disease or long duration of disease (−)
Understanding and perception of disease (+)

Source: Adapted from World Health Organization (2003). *Adherence to long-term therapies—evidence for action.* Available online at www.who.int/ chronic_conditions/en/ adherence_report.pdf. Accessed May 2005.

Notes: (+) Positive effect on adherence; (−) Negative effect on adherence.

MEDICATION-THERAPY-RELATED FACTORS

Drug therapies vary as per the duration and type of medical conditions. Each type of drug therapy contributes to different levels of patient compliance or adherence based on perceived benefits and risks of avoidance of drug therapies and relapse or onset of disease symptoms. Hopefully patients learn quickly to optimize drug therapy utilization. Drug therapy noncompliance can be viewed as an intermediate process outcome measure, reflecting the patient's preference or utility to particular medication consumption. If the risk to benefit ratio of avoiding drug therapy utilization is high then this could lead to noncompliance. In general, proven medical therapies only offer benefit to patients who actually use them and patient adherence to physicians' recommendations is the key mediator between medical practice and patient outcomes.

Interpreting adherence rates can be difficult. For example, 75 percent adherence does not necessarily mean that patients completely ignore one-fourth of recommendations received, or that 25 percent of patients never adhere. It may also mean patients may adhere to all recommendations 75 percent of the time or to somewhat less than 75 percent of recommendations an unknown percentage of the time. The interpretation of nonadherence rates in a clinical context raises important questions about the minimum level of therapeutic coverage that needs to be maintained for clinical benefit. The supposition is that 0 percent adherence results in 0 percent treatment benefit. In the highly active antiretroviral therapy, benefit is negligible unless adherence approaches 100 percent. In other conditions, benefit increases with increasing adherence, as might be the case with antihypertensive therapy. In some cases the benefit maybe limited below a certain threshold and maximal or near maximal above that threshold. For example, aspirin, if taken once a month (1 day out of 30 = 3 percent adherence), will not prevent myocardial infarction but because of the ability of aspirin to inhibit platelet aggregation and prevent clot development for a full seven days it might be highly effective if taken once a week (14 percent adherence). Thus, a 25 percent nonadherence rate may be acceptable for aspirin therapy for myocardial infarction but absolutely unacceptable for antibiotic treatment of multidrug resistant tuberculosis (Kravitz & Melnikow, 2004). Another forgiving drug, latanoprost for glaucoma, even at ill-timed doses has little impact on clinical outcomes since its activity exceeds dosing interval and appropriate therapeutic coverage is maintained. For statins, the minimum level for a positive clinical benefit (of reduction in mortality and lower risk of myocardial infarction recurrence) is taking 75 percent or more of medications (Peterson & McGhan, 2005).

The important task is establishing clinically grounded adherence models, allowing patients and clinicians to ask, "How much adherence is enough?" Further, a dynamic interaction exists between evidence about outcomes and the definition of adherence to therapy and its potential benefits for a specific clinical condition. For example, adherence to only three days of antibiotic therapy for sinusitis was very poor adherence at 30 percent, until equivalent outcomes was demonstrated between three days and ten days of antibiotic therapy for sinusitis (DiMatteo, 2004; Kravitz & Melnikow, 2004). Lack of adherence to daily antituberculosis medication led to a revised, less frequent, regimen and a new method for delivering it: directly observed therapy. Consistent performance of even "partial" adherence has led to better outcomes (Chaulk & Kazandjian, 1998). Finally, the relationship between adherence to recommended therapies and health outcomes is further complicated by evidence that those adherent with placebos have better outcomes than those who do not adhere (Epstein, 1984; Irvine et al., 1999).

Adherent individuals may have attributes leading to better health outcomes regardless of the actual benefits of therapy. In some situations greater adherence is associated with poorer outcomes. Evidence that many women were not adherent with recommended hormone replacement therapy (HRT) raised alarms (Cabana et al., 1999; Kravitz et al., 2003; Rozenberg et al., 1995) until more rigorous studies showed that HRT may cause more harm than good (Nelson, Humphrey, Nygren, Teutsch, & Allan, 2002). Further, if adverse events are avoided by nonadherence to ineffective therapies, nonadherence may be cost saving (Kravitz & Melnikow, 2004). Thus patient-centered care informing and involving patients would lead to better clinical outcomes (Greenfield, Kaplan, & Ware, 1985; Kravitz & Melnikow, 2004; Stewart et al., 2000).

There are many therapy-related factors (see Table 3.3) that affect adherence: complexity of the medical regimen, duration of treatment, previous treatment failures, frequent changes in treatment, the immediacy of beneficial effects, side effects, and the availability of medical support to deal with them. Unique characteristics of diseases and/or therapies do not outweigh the common factors affecting adherence, but rather modify their influence (WHO, 2003). Specific examples of medication-related factors affecting adherence addressed here include doses of drugs, regimen complexity, new innovative therapies with better safety and tolerability profile, longer-acting formulations, inherent drug properties, the way drugs are combined, and type of drug category.

Reduction in the number and frequency of drug doses and better knowledge about drugs may improve compliance. Observed associations with using multiple prescription and nonprescription (over the counter) medications suggest possible approaches to decreasing drug-related illness and limiting the adverse effects of hypotension in the elderly (Cohen, Rogers, Burke, Beilin, 1998). Newer drugs may be more cost effective in terms of reducing costs of inpatient care utilization. For example, evaluation in matched Medicaid patients has shown that the newer drugs, olanzapine and risperidone, in spite of their high pharmacy acquisition costs, may have optimal medication use patterns associated with greater persistence and lower inpatient service costs compared to the older antipsychotic, haloperidol (Gibson, Damler, Jackson, Wilder, & Ramsey, 2004). However, in spite of

TABLE 3.3. Medication-therapy-related factors of adherence.

Frequent doses (−)
Complex treatment regimen (−)
Adverse effects (−)
Lack of clear instructions on medication use (−)
Monotherapy (+)
Less frequent doses-few pills per day (+)
Clear instructions on treatment management (+)
New therapy (+)
Long-acting formulations (+)

Source: Adapted from World Health Organization (2003). Adherence to long-term therapies-evidence for action. Available online www.who.int/chronic_conditions/en/adherence_report.pdf. Accessed May 2005.

Notes: (+) Positive effect on adherence; (−) Negative effect on adherence.

higher adherence (as indicated by prescription refill rates) among patients on atypical antipsychotics versus traditional agents, interventions to improve adherence are needed even for atypical antipsychotics (Dolder, Lacro, Dunn, & Jeste, 2002). In another example, introduction of new thiazolidinedione therapy in a Medicaid-enrolled type 2 diabetic population was associated with significantly improved treatment adherence, persistence, and lower annual health care costs in the post-start year compared to patients starting other oral antidiabetics (Balkrishnan et al., 2004). Similarly, the new budesonide/formoterol treatment from a single inhaler reduced two-month treatment costs compared with separate inhalers, while maintaining a good control of asthma in adults (Rosenhall, Borg, Andersson, & Ericsson, 2003).

Fixed-dose combination pills and unit-of-use packaging are therapy-related interventions that are designed to simplify medication regimens and thus to potentially improve adherence. One recent systematic review of the effects of fixed-dose combination pills and unit-of-use packaging showed that the trends of improved adherence and/ or clinical outcomes reached statistical significance. However, measures of outcome were nonuniform, heterogeneous, and interpretation was further limited by methodological issues, particularly small sample size, short duration, and loss of follow-up (Connor, Rafter, & Rodgers, 2004). Extended-release (EH) formulation may ensure persistence of therapy. For example, child and adolescent Medicaid beneficiaries treated for attention-deficit/hyperactivity disorder (ADHD) showed that extended-release methylphenidate hydrochloride (ER-MPH) was associated with greater continuity of MPH treatment than IR-MPH (immediate-release methylphenidate hydrochloride) formulations. Initial selection of an ER formulation may help to prolong continuity of MPH therapy among youth Medicaid beneficiaries with ADHD (Marcus, Wan, Kemner, & Olfson, 2005).

One question would be does nonadherence vary by drug categories? Nonadherence rates were found to be equally problematic for both antipsychotic and nonpsychiatric medications (antihypertensives, antihyperlipidemics, and antidiabetics), which ranged from 52 to 64 percent in middle-aged and older patients with psychotic disorders. Interventions to improve adherence to both antipsychotic and nonpsychiatric medications are needed (Dolder, Lacro, & Jeste, 2003).

Patients may develop resistance to some drug therapies due to variance in their pharmacokinetic and pharmacodynamic properties across patients and this might require individualizing therapy, which may complicate the prognosis of the disease. Miller and Hays (2000) have noted: "For example, adherence to combination antiretroviral therapy has a strong impact on virologic response and emergence of viral resistance. Patients with suboptimal adherence may have reduced or undetectable viral loads. On the other hand, viral load may not decrease in patients with perfect adherence because of pretreatment resistance, poor drug metabolism, or other factors" (p. 177). Thus, a multidisciplinary approach with clear instructions on treatment management, involving patients, with support of health care professionals, family, and friends will optimize adherence.

PATIENT-RELATED FACTORS

Patient characteristics have been the focus of numerous investigations of adherence. Nonadherence can be of initial, intentional, or unintentional type, or of premature discontinuation. Intentional nonadherence occurs when the patient chooses not to take the drug (Elliott, Barber, & Horne, 2005; Peterson & McGhan, 2005). Initial noncompliance rates of about 13 to 25 percent are reported in terms of never filling a prescription or never claiming a filled prescription on dispensing at a pharmacy (Peterson & McGhan, 2005). Unintentional adherence occurs when the patient forgets to take the medication or inadvertently takes it incorrectly. Nonadherence can be taking medicines incorrectly (such as swallowing whole a chewable tablet), one missed dose, not taking a drug for short or long periods of time, or changing the dosing schedule or quantity (Elliott, Barber, & Horne, 2005). Delays in prescription refills also can lead to nonadherence. Premature discontinuation can be worse than initial noncompliance, especially when it carries adverse unperceived consequences such as antimicrobial resistance or rebound hypertension with beta-adrenoceptor antagonist withdrawal (Peterson & McGhan, 2005). Similarly, premature discontinuation and not treatment choice of antidepressant was associated with a high probability of relapse and recurrence in depressed Medicaid enrollees (Croghan, Melfi, Crown, & Chawla, 1998). The "variations in patients' compliance are a function of methodological and contextual factors in adherence research" (DiMatteo, 2004). In this context, it is important to examine the enabling patient attributes (that are predictors of patient adherence), which is the first step to designing effective interventions.

Socioeconomic status has not consistently been found to be an independent predictor of adherence. Some factors that are reported significant are poor socioeconomic status, poverty, illiteracy, low level of education, unemployment, lack of effective social support networks, unstable living conditions, distance from treatment center, and high cost of transport, high cost of medication, changing environmental situations, culture and lay beliefs about illness and treatment, and family dysfunction (WHO, 2003). Specifically, income and not general socioeconomic status had a positive and significant effect on adult patient adherence than on pediatric patients (DiMatteo, 2004). In several compilations, age–adherence relationship was stronger in pediatric than in adult patients, with a trend for adolescents to be less adherent than younger children at an average adherence rate of 58 percent (DiMatteo, 2004; WHO, 2003). Patient education was also found to be a positive and significant moderator of adherence, more so in chronic diseases than acute diseases. Educational efforts focusing on adolescents' attitudes toward their disease and its management, instead of predominantly on knowledge acquisition, is beneficial. Knowledge about an illness is not a correlate of nonadherence, but specific knowledge about elements of a medication regimen is, although apparently only for short-term, acute illnesses (Kirscht & Rosenstock, 1979).

Demographic variables, age, gender, education, occupation, income, marital status, race, religion, ethnic background, and urban versus rural living have not been definitely associated with adherence (Haynes, 1979; Kaplan & Simon, 1990) and have been variously shown to have some, little, or no association with adherence. Organizational variables (time spent with the doctor, continuity of care by the doctor, communication style of the doctor, and interpersonal style of the doctor) are far more important than sociodemographic variables in affecting patients' adherence (WHO, 2003). Another factor that may play an important role in adherence is ethnicity. For example, in the United States, primarily due to low health literacy, there is lack of awareness of hypertension and other cardiovascular risk factors, and low rates of control with antihypertensive drugs in the Hispanic community (Kountz, 2004). Similarly, clinicians treating schizophrenia face increasingly diverse ethnic populations. Ethnicity was a significant predictor of medication adherence following initiation on an antipsychotic medication, and patients of all ethnicities were most adherent when taking olanzapine, less adherent when taking risperidone, and least adherent when taking haloperidol (Opolka, Rascati, Brown, & Gibson, 2003).

Patient-related factors affecting adherence are forgetfulness; psychosocial stress; misunderstanding and nonacceptance of the disease; disbelief in the diagnosis; lack of perception of the health risk related to the disease; misunderstanding of treatment instructions; lack of acceptance of monitoring; low treatment expectations; lack of self-perceived need for treatment; lack of perceived effect of treatment; negative beliefs regarding the efficacy of the treatment; anxieties about possible adverse effects; low motivation; inadequate knowledge and skill in managing the disease symptoms and treatment; low attendance at follow-up, or at counseling, motivational, behavioral, or psychotherapy classes; hopelessness and negative feelings; frustration with health care providers; fear of dependence; anxiety over the complexity of the drug regimen, and feeling stigmatized by the disease (WHO, 2003).

Perceptions of personal need for medication are influenced by symptoms, expectations, experiences, and by illness cognitions. Concerns about medication typically arise from beliefs about side effects and disruption of lifestyle, and from more abstract worries about the long-term effects and dependence (WHO, 2003). Specifically in depression, patients are more likely than professionals to find the impact of spirituality, social support systems, coping strategies, life experiences, patient–provider relationships, and attributes of specific treatments important in their help-seeking behavior and treatment adherence (Cooper-Patrick et al., 1997).

Though it is a waste to health care systems, nonadherence also represents a rational choice as patients attempt to maintain their personal identity, achieve their goals, and preserve their quality of life (Bury, 1982; Charmaz, 1987; Conrad, 1985; Lambert et al., 1997; Lynn & DeGrazia, 1991; Trostle, Hauser, & Susser, 1983). Patients are often assumed to be passive, powerless, or irrational, but as consumers of many goods and services including medications, health services and pharmacy services, the majority regularly make active assessments about cost, risk, and benefit of health care (Donovan & Blake, 1992). So based on economic theory, patients can be expected to engage in utility maximization decisions.

One segment of the population which is prone to nonadherence is the elderly. The elderly represent 6.4 percent of the world's population and their numbers are increasing by 800,000 every month. This demographic transition has led to an increased prevalence of chronic conditions (Alzheimer's disease, Parkinson's disease, depression, diabetes, congestive heart failure, coronary artery disease, glaucoma, osteoarthritis, osteoporosis, and others) that are particularly common in the elderly.

Many elderly patients present with multiple chronic diseases, which require complex long-term treatment to prevent frailty and disability. Furthermore, the elderly are the greatest consumers of prescription drugs. In developed countries, people over sixty years old consume approximately 50 percent of all prescription medicines (as much as three times more per capita than the general population) and are responsible for 60 percent of medication-related costs even though they represent only 12 to 18 percent of the population in these countries. In the elderly, failure to adhere to medical recommendations and treatment has been found to increase the likelihood of therapeutic failure, and to be responsible for unnecessary complications, leading to increased spending on health care, as well as to disability and early death. Age-related alterations in pharmacokinetics and pharmacodynamics make this population even more vulnerable to problems resulting from nonadherence (WHO, 2003).

Predictors that may predispose the elderly to medication nonadherence include demographics that can predict nonadherence risk, specific disease states, like cardiovascular diseases and depression, multiple comorbidities, complex medical regimens, a decline in functional abilities (Conrad, 1985), poor communication between health professionals and the elderly (Morrow, Leirer, & Sheikh, 1988), the presence of cognitive and functional (vision, hearing) impairment, and/or inadequate or marginal health literacy, and disability. Social and financial resources may also complicate the ability of older adults to adhere to pharmacologic prescriptions. The most practical method of medication adherence assessment for most elderly patients may be through patient or caregiver interview using open-ended, nonthreatening, and nonjudgmental questions. Medication adherence requires a working relationship between a patient or caregiver and prescriber that values open, honest discussion about medications, that is, the administration schedule, intended benefits, adverse effects and costs (MacLaughlin et al., 2005). Especially, out-of-pocket costs and inadequate prescription coverage are common among elderly patients with comorbid diseases, although drug coverage may protect patients from this increased risk (Piette, Wagner, Potter, & Schillinger, 2004; Piette, Heisler, & Wagner, 2004a). Many chronically ill adults frequently cut back on medications by being selective about the treatments they forego due to economic constraints (Piette, Heisler, & Wagner, 2004b).

In summary, patient-related factors represent the resources, knowledge, attitudes, beliefs, perceptions, and expectations of the patient (see Table 3.4). Knowing the limited role of demographics (age, gender, patient education, and socioeconomic status) is important. The factors that can have greater effect on adherence are the ones most amenable to change. These include treating anxiety and depression, offering practical and emotional support, and considering income, which would improve adherence and patient's quality of life

TABLE 3.4. Patient-related (including socioeconomic-related) factors of adherence.

Patient related
Forgetfulness (−)
Inadequate knowledge and self-management skills in managing disease symptoms and treatment (−)
Misunderstanding instructions of how to take medications (−)
Anxieties about possible adverse effects (−)
Lack of self-perceived need for treatment (−)
Psychosocial distress, depression (−)
Low motivation (−)
Ethnicity (+)
Belief in efficacy of treatment (+)
Motivation (+)
Perception of health risk related to the disease (+)
Socioeconomic
Long distance from treatment setting (−)
Low socioeconomic status (−)
Illiteracy (−)
High cost of medication (−)
Family support (+)

Source: Adapted from World Health Organization (2003). *Adherence to long-term therapies—evidence for action.* Available online www.who.int/chronic_conditions/en/adherence_report.pdf. Accessed May, 2005.

Notes: (+) Positive effect on adherence; (−) Negative effect on adherence.

(Chesney, Chrisman, Luftey, Pescosolido, & Anderson, 1999; DiMatteo, Lepper, & Croghan, 2000; Lustman et al., 1995; Rosenhall et al., 2003; Takiya, Peterson, & Finley, 2004; Ziegelstein et al., 2000). Patients' knowledge and beliefs about their illness, motivation to manage it, confidence (self-efficacy) in their ability to engage in illness management behaviors, and expectations regarding the outcome of treatment and the consequences of poor adherence, interact in ways not yet fully understood to influence adherence behavior. Specifically, patient's motivation to adhere to prescribed treatment is influenced by the value placed on following the regimen (cost-benefit ratio) and the degree of confidence in being able to follow it. Building on a patient's intrinsic motivation by increasing the perceived importance of adherence, and strengthening confidence by building self-management skills, are behavioral treatment targets that must be addressed concurrently with biomedical ones if overall adherence is to be improved (WHO, 2003). Thus, strategies to improve adherence will need to be multidimensional, including improvements in pharmacy services that consider age-related factors (e.g., declining cognitive and physical functions) as well as a variety of environmental and social factors (Donovan & Blake, 1992).

HEALTH PROFESSIONAL ATTRIBUTES AND HEALTH SYSTEM FACTORS

Health Professional Attributes

Poor adherence is a remedial problem in health care quality and its improvement and accountability offer shared opportunities for providers and patients. Adherence is not just for patients: when it comes to performing recommended practice behaviors, physicians have issues of their own. Numerous studies have shown that physician compliance with proven beneficial practices is far from optimal. Systematic approaches to improving prescribing practices are increasing (Wahl et al., 2005).

Physicians' attributes and practice style are reported to influence patients' adherence to treatment in diabetes, hypertension, and heart disease patients. Other provider predictors of patient adherence (general and specific to medication, exercise, and diet recommendations) were physician job satisfaction (general adherence), number of patients seen per week (medication), scheduling a follow-up appointment (medication), tendency to answer patients' questions (exercise), number of tests ordered (diet), seriousness of illness (diet), physician specialty (medication, diet), and patient health distress (medication, exercise) (DiMatteo et al., 1993). Physician follow-up communication style and patient satisfaction have both been shown to be predictive of better medication adherence (Bultman & Svarstad, 2000; Hall, Roter, & Katz, 1988). For example, patients initiated hormone replacement therapy (HRT) in 39.2 percent of physician visits in which it was discussed. Patients with diabetes were less likely to discuss HRT. Increasing years of physician residency was associated with decreased discussion of HRT. When physicians were similar in age and training, male physicians discussed HRT significantly more often than did female physicians (Huston, Sleath, & Rubin, 2001).

The quality of the interactive process has also been reported to be critical to the establishment and shaping of the therapeutic patient–physician relationship, which is related to physician gender. An analysis of the literature on communication differences between physicians of different genders indicates that female physicians facilitate and show a greater affinity for collaborative patient–physician relationship models than do their male colleagues, spend more time with their patients, are more likely to engage their patients in discussions of their social and psychological factors, and deal more often with feelings and emotions (Roter & Hall, 1998).

About one-third of chronically ill adults who underuse prescription medication because of the cost never talk with clinicians in advance, and many never raise this issue at all. Clinicians should take a more proactive role in identifying and assisting patients who have problems paying for prescription drugs (Piette, Heisler, & Wagner, 2004a). Predictors of patient participation in comprehensive cardiac rehabilitation program that reduces mortality and morbidity were as follows: physician's endorsement of the effectiveness of such a program, and active physician referral. Further, being educated, married, having high self-efficacy, travel accessible programs or no experience of guilt over family obligations were other predictors of patient participation. Women were less often referred and participated less often even after referral. Many of the observed predictors are potentially modifiable by health professionals (Jackson, Leclerc, Erskine, & Linden, 2005). One review showed that cultural competence training showed promise as a strategy for improving the knowledge, attitudes, and skills of health professionals (Beach et al., 2005).

Doctors do not suspect frequently that their patients are not taking their drugs exactly as prescribed. Patients rarely volunteer this information to their doctor, and doctors do not often explicitly ask (Rogers & Bullman, 1995), so adherence often goes undetected. On the other hand, prescribing decision related overuse and underuse can also lead to nonadherence. Take for example, a controlled study of the effects of New York state physician surveillance requirements through a Triplicate Prescription Program (TPP) on indicators of problematic/nonproblematic benzodiazepine use in a Medicaid population. State-mandated physician surveillance dramatically reduced benzodiazepine use with limited substitution of alternative drugs, lowered rates of possible abuse, but also severely limited nonproblematic benzodiazepine use (Ross-Degnan et al., 2004). Another example by in patients with coronary artery disease. High cholesterol, the 3-hydroxy-3-methylglutaryl coenzyme A reductase inhibitors (or "statins") have been shown to reduce overall mortality in primary and secondary prevention of coronary artery disease. The National Cholesterol Education Program expert panel's guidelines (Adult Treatment Panel III) recommend evaluation and treatment of high cholesterol based on stratification of patients according to cardiovascular risk. For all patients at a tertiary medical center, overuse of statin therapy was found among 69 percent of patients undergoing primary prevention and among 47 percent of patients undergoing secondary prevention. Among patients with coronary heart disease who were not taking statins, 88 percent were undertreated. Monitoring of liver function varied widely and did not correlate with the risk of adverse events secondary to statin use. Overtreatment and undertreatment for hyperlipidemia have been frequently reported (Abookire, Karson, Fiskio, & Bates, 2001).

Studies have shown that concomitant complex therapies may also affect provider's medication prescribing decisions. Effective therapy for chronic illness requires daily medication adherence (DMA) for prolonged periods. Patients with more concurrently prescribed medicines had higher DMA and better, though suboptimal, refill persistence (RP), even after adjusting for demographic factors and cardiovascular comorbidity. Physicians should not be deterred from initiating statin therapy by a patient's medical regimen complexity but should be alert for lack of therapy persistence, particularly in younger and healthier patients (Grant, O'Leary, Weilburg, Singer, & Meigs, 2004). Audit, decision support systems, and feedback can continue to be widely used as a strategy to improve professional practice performance compared with guidelines. The absolute effects of these strategies are likely to be larger when baseline adherence to recommended practice is low and recommendations are applicable and they are tolerated by the patient population they serve (Jamtvedt et al., 2003). Patient recall and comprehension also were associated with physicians' communication (Stewart, 1996; Cruz & Pincus, 2002). Associations have been observed between physicians' communicative skills and patients' satisfaction, patients' adherence to treatment recommendations, treatment outputs, and patients' willingness to file malpractice claims. The research has also shown that primary care physicians can be more responsive to patients' concerns without lengthening visits (Cruz & Pincus, 2002).

Pharmacists and other nonphysicians have always been part of the system of checks and balances in health care delivery. As the provision of health services changes, pharmacists are well positioned to intervene in patient care and have documented and demonstrated that the value of pharmacy services goes beyond dispensing to include provision of cognitive services such as compliance programs, screening services, glucose monitoring, and disease management programs (Mullins, Baldwin, & Perfetto, 1996). Pharmacy practice and provider characteristics may be facilitators or barriers to providing effective adherence enhancing interventions to patients. One study has reported that antidepressant medication telemonitoring by community pharmacists significantly and positively affected patient feedback and collaboration with pharmacists (Rickles et al., 2005). Community pharmacies in eight states showed that pharmacist counseling varied significantly according to the intensity of state regulation, pharmacy business, and age of the responsible pharmacist. While pharmacy type was unrelated to counseling, business reduced the odds of any pharmacist talk, oral information giving, and assessment of understanding. Frequency of information provision increased from 40 to 94 percent as states' counseling regulations increased in intensity. These results can be used by policymakers and individual practitioners who are in a position to improve upon this important element of patient adherence care (Svarstad, Bultman, & Mount, 2004).

Health professional training should not be discounted as a predictor of adherence to guideline-based prescribing which in turn impacts patient adherence. It is well known that health professionals' advice to patients on behavior has been less than optimal. Despite national guidelines, studies across the country have shown that many physicians do not regularly engage in assisting their patients with tobacco cessation behaviors (Gill, Diamond, Leone, Pellini, & Wender, 2004). For example only 60 percent of physicians were aware of coverage of nicotine-replacement pharmacotherapies for Medicaid enrollees (Mc-Menamin, Halpin, Ibrahim, & Orleans, 2004). Specifically, formal training in smoking cessation has had a significant impact on physician self-efficacy related to smoking cessation and has implications for their ability to counsel parents about smoking cessation (Cabana et al., 2004). Similarly, willingness to give time for patient compliance enhancing strategies by health professionals is an important attribute that could promote compliance behavior in patients.

Health-System-Related Factors

Access to medications is necessary but insufficient in itself for the successful treatment of disease. The policies and procedures of the health system also control access to, and the quality of care provided (WHO, 2003). For example, after implementation of a cost-containment measure (the preferred drug list), Medicaid patients were more likely to discontinue filling prescriptions for antihypertensive medication, which in turn adversely affected adherence (Wilson, Axelsen, & Tang, 2005). Hence important health system variables that affect adherence include the availability and accessibility of services, support for patient education, data collection and information management, provision of feedback to patients and health care providers, community supports available to patients, and the training provided to health service providers. Through these system variables, the health care delivery system has great potential to facilitate the patient's adherence behavior, which may not be possible through the provision of prescription drug benefit coverage alone. Systems direct providers' schedules, dictate appointment lengths and duration of treatment, allocate resources, set fee structures, and establish organizational priorities for continuity of care, information sharing, and level of communication with patients. Providers often report that they have insufficient time to address adherence behavior adequately. Many health systems lack financial coverage for patient counseling and education, which leaves out many adherence-focused interventions. Increased demands upon providers have been associated with decreased patient adherence. Patients demonstrate better adherence when they receive care from the same provider over time. The ability of clinics and pharmacies to share information regarding patients' behavior toward prescription refills also has the potential to improve adherence. Ongoing communication efforts (e.g., telephone reminders) that keep the patient engaged in health care may be the simplest and most cost-effective strategy for improving adherence (WHO, 2003). For example, persistence with lipid-lowering agents is low among the elderly managed care enrollees regardless of scope of drug benefit coverage or the drug class will require a multifaceted approach (Abughosh, Kogut, Andrade, Larrat, & Gurwitz, 2004).

Thus, factors related to health professionals and health care systems (see Table 3.5) are important determinants of patient adherence. Positive relationships have been reported between treatment adherence and provider communication styles characterized by providing information, "positive talk," asking patients specific questions about adherence, clarity of diagnostic and treatment advice in the short-term but not long-term regimens, continuity of care (follow-up), warmth and empathy of the clinician, active patient involvement in their care process and patient satisfaction. Providers who share information, build partnerships, and provide emotional support have better patient outcomes than the patients of providers who do not interact in this manner. There is evidence that, in practice, health professionals give limited information, lack skills in motivational enhancement, and lack knowledge and experience frustration in teaching patients behavioral skills. More structured and thoughtful interactions between provider and patient are essential for improvements in adherence.

Relatively little research has been conducted on the effects of a health care professional team and system-related factors on adherence. The factors that have a negative effect on adherence include poorly developed health services with inadequate or nonexistent reimbursement by health insurance plans, poor medication distribution systems, lack of knowledge and training for health care providers on managing chronic diseases, overworked health care providers, lack of incentives and feedback on performance to providers, short consultations, poor capacity of the system to educate patients and provide follow-up, and inability to establish community support and self-management capacity (Hall, Roter, & Katz, 1988; WHO, 2003).

TABLE 3.5. Health professional attributes and health-system-related factors of adherence.

Health professional attributes

    Short consultations (−)

    Poor relationship between patient and physician (−)

    Lack of knowledge and training of health professionals about treatment management (−)

    Inadequate understanding of the disease (−)

    Lack of time (−)

    Good relationship between patient and health professionals (+)

Health system factors

    Poor implementation of educational interventions (−)

    Support for providers to engage in patient education (+)

    Availability and accessibility of services (+)

    Organizational priorities (−)

    Reimbursement to provider for cognitive services rendered to patients

---

Source: Adapted from World Health Organization (2003). *Adherence to long-term therapies—evidence for action.* Available online www.who.int/chronic_conditions/en/adherence_report.pdf. Accessed May 2005.

Notes: (+) Positive effect on adherence; (−) negative effect on adherence.

Health care providers should be able to assess the patient's readiness to adhere, provide advice on how to do it, and follow up the patient's progress at every contact. Health providers can have a significant impact by assessing risk of nonadherence and delivering interventions to optimize adherence. To make this practice a reality, practitioners must have access to specific training in adherence management, and the systems in which they work must design and support delivery systems that respect this objective.

Governmental programs, for example, systems like Medicare began providing prescription drug coverage (Part D) for the elderly beginning January 2006, as part of the Medicare Prescription Drug, Improvement, and Modernization Act of 2003. The act also includes a provision for high-risk targeted beneficiaries to receive Medication Therapy Management Services (MTMS), which may be furnished by a pharmacist or other provider to Part D eligible Medicare enrollees with two or more chronic conditions, taking multiple medications and who are likely to incur annual expenses beyond the level specified by the Secretary of the Department of Health and Human Services. Further, effective from January 1, 2006, a set of three Health Insurance Portability and Accountability Act (HIPAA)-compliant American Medical Association (AMA) Current Procedural Terminology (CPT) codes was made available. These codes are for pharmacists to use for billing third-party payors (any health plan that provides a benefit for MTMS, including those covered under the new Medicare Part D Prescription Drug Benefit). Patients will benefit from having uniform, reliable, documentation of the valuable professional services that they receive from pharmacists regarding appropriate medication therapy use (ASHP, 2005). Thus, these incentives can encourage providers to deliver adherence education to patients. In conclusion, there is an ongoing need to simultaneously address three topics: knowledge (information on adherence and comprehensive adherence interventions that are mutually beneficial for patients and providers (Gill et al., 2004)), thinking (the clinical decision-making process), and action (effective behavioral tools for health professionals). This will lead to ongoing dynamic implementation of effective adherence assessments and interventions in health care systems (WHO, 2003).

CONCLUSIONS AND FUTURE DIRECTIONS

The structure and demand of various drug therapies is heterogeneous across different medical conditions. Well-defined multidisciplinary patient interventions, explaining use of medications, continuing tailored education, monitoring of the treatment regimen, minimizing clinical side effects, reminding and motivating patients to adhere with the regimen, and finally promoting communication between providers and patients is important in chronic disease management and formulation of guidelines-based therapy to ensure maximum therapy effectiveness.

The lack of a match between patient readiness and the practitioner's intervention means that treatments are frequently prescribed to patients who are not ready to follow them. The goal of the providers should not to be to pressurize patients into compliance but to make sure that the patient understands the consequences either way, and to address any medical, social, and emotional factors that undermine the patient's will to adhere. Patient participation can be a powerful driver and can modify physician behavior to improve health outcomes and quality of care. To improve adherence, a continuous and dynamic process, more studies must be conducted (DiMatteo, 2004).

Plans for medication adherence should consider modifiable predictors of medical condition, medication, patient, provider- and system-related factors of nonadherence. These factors are targets for interventions, which may be combined when necessary to optimize adherence (Krueger, Felkey, & Berger, 2003; Nichols-English & Poirier, 2000). Mixed comprehensive interventions that included educational, behavioral (to develop self-management skills), and affective elements were more effective than single-focus interventions (Roter et al., 1998). Systems that accurately assess and actively consider the determinants of adherence, along with advances in biomedical technology are imperative. A stronger coordinated commitment to a multidisciplinary multilevel approach targeting many factors is needed from patients, health professionals, researchers, health planners, and policymakers in health care systems to effectively improve medication adherence, to reduce costs, and improve health outcomes.

REFERENCES

Abookire, S. A., Karson, A. S., Fiskio, J., & Bates, D. W. (2001). Use and monitoring of "statin" lipid-lowering drugs compared with guidelines. *Arch Intern Med, 161*(1): 53-58.

Abughosh, S. M., Kogut, S. J., Andrade, S. E., Larrat, P., & Gurwitz, J. H. (2004). Persistence with lipid-lowering therapy: Influence of the type of lipid-lowering agent and drug benefit plan option in elderly patients. *J Manag Care Pharm, 10*(5): 404-411.

Aday, L. A., Begley, C. E., Lairson, D. R., & Balkrishnan, R. (2004). *Evaluating the healthcare system: Effectiveness, efficiency, and equity.* Chicago, IL: Health Administration Press, pp. 93-120.

Andersen R., & Newman, J. F. (1973). Societal and individual determinants of Med Care utilization in the United States. *Milbank Mem Fund Q Health Soc, 51*(1): 95-124.

ASHP. Professional Service Billing Codes Approved for Pharmacists–American Society of Health system pharmacist website Release dated July 7, 2005; http://www.ashp.org/news/ShowArticle.cfm?id=11615 accessed July 2005.

Balkrishnan R. (2005). The importance of medication adherence in improving chronic-disease related outcomes: What we know and what we need to further know. *Med Care, 43*(6): 517-520.

Balkrishnan, R., Rajagopalan, R., Camacho, F. T., Huston, S. A., Murray, F. T., & Anderson, R. T. (2003). Predictors of medication adherence and associated health care costs in an older population with type 2 diabetes mellitus: A longitudinal cohort study. *Clin Ther, 25*: 2958-2971.

Barber, N. (2002). Should we consider non-compliance a medical error? *Qual Saf Health Care, 11*: 81-84.

Beach, M. C., Price, E. G., Gary, T. L., Robinson, K. A., Gozu, A., Palacio, A., Smarth, C., Jenckes, M. W., Feuerstein, C., Bass, E. B., Powe, N. R., & Cooper, L. A. (2005). Cultural competence: A systematic review of health care provider educational interventions. *Med Care, 43*(4): 356-373.

Bender, B. G., & Rand, C. (2004). Medication non-adherence and asthma treatment cost. *Curr Opin Allergy Clin Immunol, 4*: 191-195.

Bowen, D. J., Helmes, A., & Lease, E. (2001). Predicting compliance: How are we doing? In Burke, L. E., & Ockene, I. S. (Eds.), *Compliance in Healthcare and Research* (pp. 25-41). Armonk, NY: Futura.

Boyd, J. R., Covington, T. R., Stanaszek, W. F., & Coussons, R. T. (1974). Drug defaulting: Part I. Determinants of compliance. *Am J Hospital Pharmacy, 31*: 362.

Bultman, D. C., & Svarstad, B. L. (2000). Effects of physician communication style on client medication beliefs and adherence with antidepressant treatment. *Patient Educ Couns, 40*(2): 173-185.

Bury, M. (1982). Chronic illness as biographical disruption. *Sociol Health Illness, 4*: 167-182.

Cabana, M. D., Rand, C., Slish, K., Nan, B., Davis, M. M., & Clark, N. (2004). Pediatrician self-efficacy for counseling parents of asthmatic children to quit smoking. *Pediatrics, 113*(1 Pt 1): 78-81.

Cabana, M. D., Rand, C. S., Powe, N. R., Wu, A. W., Wilson, M. H., Abboud, P. A., & Rubin, H. R. (1999). Why don't physicians follow clinical practice guidelines? A framework for improvement. *JAMA, 282*: 1458-1465.

Charmaz K. (1987). Struggling for a self: Identity levels of the chronically ill. In Roth, J., & Conrad, P., (Eds.), *Research in the sociology of health care*. Vol. 6. *The experience and management of chronic illness* (pp. 283-321). Greenwich, CT: JAI Press.

Chaulk, C. P., & Kazandjian, V. A. (1998). Directly observed therapy for treatment completion of pulmonary tuberculosis: Consensus Statement of the Public Health Tuberculosis Guidelines Panel. *JAMA, 279*: 943-948.

Chesney, M., Chrisman, N. J., Luftey, K., Pescosolido, B., & Anderson, N. (1999). Not what the doctor ordered: Challenges individuals face in adhering to medical advice/treatment. *Congressional briefing*. Washington, DC: Consortium of Social Science Associations.

Cohen, I., Rogers, P., Burke, V., & Beilin, L. J. (1998). Predictors of medication use, compliance and symptoms of hypotension in a community-based sample of elderly men and women. *J Clin Pharm Ther, 23*(6): 423-432.

Connor, J., Rafter, N., & Rodgers, A. (2004). Do fixed-dose combination pills or unit-of-use packaging improve adherence? A systematic review. *Bull World Health Organ, 82*(12): 935-939.

Conrad, P. (1985). The meaning of medications: Another look at compliance. *Soc Sci Med, 20*: 29-37.

Cooper-Patrick, L., Powe, N. R., Jenckes, M. W., Gonzales, J. J., Levine, D. M., & Ford, D. E. (1997). Identification of patient attitudes and preferences regarding treatment of depression. *J Gen Intern Med, 12*(7): 431-438.

Croghan, T. W., Melfi, C. A., Crown, W. E., & Chawla, A. (1998). Cost-effectiveness of antidepressant medications. *J Ment Health Policy Econ, 1*(3): 109-117.

Cruz M., & Pincus, H. A. (2002). Research on the influence that communication in psychiatric encounters has on treatment. *Psychiatr Serv, 53*(10): 1253-1265.

DiMatteo, R. (2004). Variations in patients' adherence to medical recommendations: A quantitative review of 50 years of research. *Med Care, 42*: 200-209.

DiMatteo, M. R., Giordani, P. J., Lepper, H. S., & Groghan, T. W. (2002). Patient adherence and medical treatment outcomes: A meta-analysis. *Med Care, 40*: 794-811.

DiMatteo, M. R., Lepper, H. S., & Croghan, T. W. (2000). Depression is a risk factor for noncompliance with medical treatment: A meta-analysis of the effects of anxiety and depression on patient adherence. *Arch Intern Med, 160*: 2101-2107.

DiMatteo, M. R., Sherbourne, C. D., Hays, R. D., Ordway, L., Kravitz, R. L., McGlynn, E. A., Kaplan, S., & Rogers, W. H. (1993). Physicians' characteristics influence patients' adherence to medical treatment: Results from the Medical Outcomes Study. *Health Psychol, 12*(2): 93-102.

Dolder, C. R., Lacro, J. P., Dunn, L. B., & Jeste, D. V. (2002). Antipsychotic medication adherence: Is there a difference between typical and atypical agents? *Am J Psychiatry, 159*: 103-108.

Dolder, C. R., Lacro, J. P., & Jeste, D. V. (2003). Adherence to antipsychotic and nonpsychiatric medications in middle-aged and older patients with psychotic disorders. *Psychosom Med, 65*(1): 156-162.

Donovan, J., & Blake, D. R. (1992). Patient non-compliance: Deviance or reasoned decision-making. *Soc Sci Med, 34*: 507-513.

Elliott, R. A., Barber, N., & Horne, R. (2005). Cost-effectiveness of adherence-enhancing interventions: A quality assessment of the evidence. *Ann Pharmacother, 39*(3): 508-515.

Epstein, L. H. (1984). The direct effects of compliance on health outcome. *Health Psychol, 3*: 385-393.

Fincham, J. E., ed. (1995). *Advancing prescription medicine compliance: New paradigms, new practices.* Binghamton, NY: Pharmaceutical Product Press, an imprint of The Haworth Press Inc.

Gibson, P. J., Damler, R., Jackson, E. A., Wilder, T., & Ramsey, J. L. (2004). The impact of olanzapine, risperidone, or haloperidol on the cost of schizophrenia care in a Medicaid population. *Value in Health, 7*(1): 22-35.

Gill, J. M., Diamond, J. J., Leone, F. T., Pellini, B., & Wender, R. C. (2004). Do physicians in Delaware follow national guidelines for tobacco counseling? *Del Med J, 76*(8): 297-308.

Grant, R. W., O'Leary, K. M., Weilburg, J. B., Singer, D. E., & Meigs, J. B. (2004). Impact of concurrent medication use on statin adherence and refill persistence. *Arch Intern Med, 164*(21): 2343-2348.

Greenfield, S., Kaplan, S., & Ware, J. E. (1985). Expanding patient involvement in care: Effects on patient outcomes. *Ann Intern Med, 102*: 520-528.

Hall, J. A., Roter, D. L., & Katz, N. R. (1988). Meta-analysis of correlates of provider behavior in medical encounters. *Med Care, 26*: 657.

Haynes, R. B. (1979). Determinants of compliance: The disease and the mechanics of treatment. Baltimore, MD: Johns Hopkins University Press.

Haynes, R. B., McDonald, H., Garg, A. X., & Montague, P. (2002). Interventions for helping patients to follow prescriptions for medications. *Cochrane Database Syst Rev, (2):* CD000011.

Huston, S., Sleath, B., & Rubin, R. H. (2001). Physician gender and hormone replacement therapy discussion. *J Wom Health Gender-Based Med, 10*(3): 279-287.

Irvine, J., Brian, B., Smith, J., Jandciu, S., Paquette, M., Cairns, J. et al. (1999). Poor adherence to placebo or amiodarone therapy predicts mortality: Results from the CAMIAT study. *Psychosom Med, 61*: 566-575.

Jackson, L., Leclerc, J., Erskine, Y., & Linden, W. (2005). Getting the most out of cardiac rehabilitation: A review of referral and adherence predictors. *Heart, 91*(1): 10-14.

Jamtvedt, G., Young, J. M., Kristoffersen, D. T., Thomson O'Brien, M. A., & Oxman, A. D. (2003). Audit and feedback: Effects on professional practice and health care outcomes. *Cochrane Database Syst Rev, (3):* CD000259.

Kaplan, R. M., & Simon, H. J. (1990). Compliance in med care: Reconsideration of self-predictions. *Ann Behav Med, 12*: 66-71.

Kirscht, J., & Rosenstock, I. (1979). Patient's problems in following recommendations of health experts. In Stone, C. (Eds.), *Health psychology* (pp. 189-216). San Francisco: Jossey-Bass.

Kountz, D. S. (2004). Hypertension in ethnic populations: Tailoring treatments. *Clin Cornerstone, 6*(3): 39-46; discussion 47-48.

Kravitz, R. L., Bell, R. A., Azari, R., Kelly-Reif, S., Krupat, E., & Thom, D. H. (2003). Direct observation of requests for clinical services in office practice: What do patients want and do they get it? *Arch Intern Med, 28*(163): 1673-1681.

Kravitz, R. L., & Melnikow J. (2004). Medical adherence research: Time for a change in direction? *Med Care, 42*(3): 197-199.

Krueger, K. P., Felkey, B. G., & Berger, B. A. (2003). Improving adherence and persistence: A review and assessment of interventions and description of steps toward a national adherence initiative. *J Am Pharm Assoc, 43*(6): 665.

Lambert, B. L., Street, R. L., Cegala, D. J., Smith, D. H., Kurtz, S., & Schofield, T. L. (1997). Provider-patient communication, patient-centered care, and the mangle of practice. *Health Commun, 9:* 27-43.

Leventhal, H., & Cameron, L. (1994). Persuasion and health attitudes. In Shavitt, S. & B. T. C. (Eds.), *Persuasion* (pp. 219-249). Boston: Allyn & Bacon.

Lustman, P. J. et al. (1995). Effects of alprazolam on glucose regulation in diabetes. Results of double-blind, placebo-controlled trial. *Diabetes Care, 18:* 1133-1139.

Lynn, J., & DeGrazia D. (1991). An outcomes model of medical decision making. *Theor Med Bioeth, 12:* 325-343.

Marcus, S. C., Wan, G. J., Kemner, J. E., & Olfson, M. (2005). Continuity of methylphenidate treatment for attention-deficit/hyperactivity disorder. *Arch Pediatr Adolesc Med, 159*(6): 572-578.

MacLaughlin, E. J., Raehl, C. L., Treadway, A. K., Sterling, T. L., Zoller, D. P., & Bond C. A. (2005). Assessing medication adherence in the elderly: Which tools to use in clinical practice? *Drugs Aging, 22*(3): 231-255.

McDonald, H. P., Garg, A. X., & Haynes, R. B. (2002) Interventions to enhance patient adherence to medication prescriptions: Scientific review. *JAMA, 288*(22): 2868-2879.

McMenamin, S. B., Halpin, H. A., Ibrahim, J. K., & Orleans, C. T. (2004). Physician and enrollee knowledge of Medicaid coverage for tobacco dependence treatments. *Am J Prev Med, 26*(2): 99-104.

Merriam-Webster. Merriam-Webster Online Dictionary URL: http://www.m-w.com/cgi-bin/dictionary?book=Dictionary&va=compliance. Accessed July 23, 2005.

Mihalko, S. L., Brenes, G. A., Farmer, D. F., Katula, J. A., Balkrishnan, R., & Bowen, D. J. (2004). Challenges and innovations in enhancing adherence. *Control Clin Trials, 25:* 447-457.

Miller, L. G., & Hays, R. D. (2000). Adherence to combination antiretroviral therapy: Synthesis of the literature and clinical implications. *AIDS Read, 10*(3): 177-185.

Morrow, D., Leirer, V., & Sheikh J. (1988). Adherence and medication instructions. Review and recommendations. *J Am Geriatr Soc, 36*(12): 1147-1160.

Mullins, C. D., Baldwin, R., & Perfetto, E. M. (1996). What are outcomes? *J Am Pharm Assoc, NS36*(1): 39-49.

Murray, M. D., Morrow, D. G., Weiner, M., Clark, D. O., Tu, W., Deer, M. M., Brater, D. C., & Weinberger, M. (2004). A conceptual framework to study medication adherence in older adults. *Am J Geriatr Pharmacother, 2*(1): 36-43.

Nelson, H. D., Humphrey, L. L., Nygren, P., Teutsch, S. M., & Allan, J. D. (2002). Postmenopausal hormone replacement therapy: Scientific review. *JAMA, 288:* 872-881.

Nichols-English G., & Poirier S. (2000) Optimizing adherence to pharmaceutical care plans. *J Am Pharm Assoc, 40*(4): 475-485.

Oldridge, N. B. (2001). Future directions: What paths do researchers need to take? What needs to be done to improve multi-level compliance? In Burke, L. E., & Ockene, I. S. (Eds.), *Compliance in healthcare and research* (pp. 331-347). Armonk, NY: Futura.

Opolka, J. L., Rascati, K. L., Brown, C. M., & Gibson, P. J. (2003). Role of ethnicity in predicting antipsychotic medication adherence. *Ann Pharmacother, 37*(5): 625-630.

Peterson, A. M., & McGhan, W. F. (2005). Pharmacoeconomic impact of non-compliance with statins. *Pharmacoeconomics, 23*(1): 13-25.

Piette, J. D., Heisler, M., & Wagner, T. H. (2004a). Cost-related medication underuse: Do patients with chronic illnesses tell their doctors? *Arch Intern Med, 164*(16): 1749-1755.

Piette, J. D., Heisler, M., & Wagner, T. H. (2004b). Cost-related medication underuse among chronically ill adults: The treatments people forgo, how often, and
who is at risk. *Am J Public Health, 94*(10): 1782-1787.
Piette, J. D., Wagner, T. H., Potter, M. B., & Schillinger, D. (2004). Health insurance
status, cost-related medication underuse, and outcomes among diabetes patients
in three systems of care. *Med Care, 42*(2): 102-109.
Rand, C. S. (1993). Measuring adherence with therapy for chronic diseases: Implications for the treatment of heterozygous familial hypercholesterolemia. *Am J
Cardiol, 72:* 68D-74D.
Rickles, N. M., Svarstad, B. L., Statz-Paynter, J. L., Taylor, L. V., & Kobak, K. A.
(2005). Pharmacist telemonitoring of antidepressant use: Effects on pharmacist-
patient collaboration. *J Am Pharm Assoc, 45*(3): 344-353.
Rogers, P. G., & Bullman, W. R. (1995). Prescription medicine compliance: A review of the baseline of knowledge. A report of the National Council on Patient
Information and Education. *J Pharmacoepidemiology, 2:* 3.
Rosenhall, L., Borg, S., Andersson, F., & Ericsson, K. (2003). Budesonide/formoterol
in a single inhaler (Symbicort) reduces healthcare costs compared with separate inhalers in the treatment of asthma over 12 months. *Int J Clin Pract, 57*(8): 662-667.
Ross-Degnan, D., Simoni-Wastila, L., Brown, J. S., Gao, X., Mah, C., Cosler, L. E.
et al. (2004). A controlled study of the effects of state surveillance on indicators
of problematic and non-problematic benzodiazepine use in a Medicaid population. *Int J Psychiatry Med, 34*(2): 103-123.
Roter, D. L., & Hall, J. A. (1998). Why physician gender matters in shaping the phy-
sician-patient relationship. *J Womens Health, 7*(9): 1093-1097.
Roter, D. L., Hall, J. A., Merisca, R., Nordstrom, B., Cretin, D., Svarstad, B. (1998).
Effectiveness of interventions to improve patient compliance: A meta-analysis.
Med Care, 36(8): 1138-1161.
Rozenberg, S., Vandromme, J., Kroll, M., Pastijn A, & Liebens F. (1995). Compli-
ance to hormone replacement therapy. *Int J Fertil Menopausal Stud, 40*(1): 23-32.
Sackett, D. L., Haynes, R. B., eds. (1976). *Compliance with therapeutic regimens.*
Baltimore, MD: Johns Hopkins University Press.
Singh, N., Squier, C., Sivek, C., Wagener, M., Nguyen, H., & Yu, V. L. (1996). De-
terminants of compliance with antiretroviral therapy in patients with human immunodeficiency virus: Prospective assessment with implications for enhancing
compliance. *AIDS Care, 8:* 261-269.
Sokol, M. C., McGuigan, K. A., Verbrugge, R. R., Epstein, & R. S. (2005). Impact of
medication adherence on hospitalization risk and healthcare cost. *Med Care,
43*(6): 521-530.
Smith, M. C. (1996a). Determinants of medication use. In Smith, M. C. & Wertheimer, A. I. (Eds), *Social and behavioral aspects of pharmaceutical care* (pp. 295-
322). Binghamton, NY: Pharmaceutical Product Press, an imprint of The
Haworth Press.
Smith, M. C. (1996b). Predicting and Detecting Noncompliance. In Smith, M. C. &
Wertheimer, A. I. (Eds.), *Social and behavioral aspects of pharmaceutical care*
(pp. 323-350). Binghamton, NY: Pharmaceutical Product Press, an imprint of
The Haworth Press Inc.

Stewart, M., Brown, J. B., Donner, A., McWhinney, I. R., Oates, J., Weston, W. W., & Jordan, J. (2000). The impact of patient-centered care on outcomes. *J Fam Pract, 49:* 796-804.

Stewart, M. A. (1996). Effective physician-patient communication and health outcomes: A review. *Can Med Assoc J, 152:* 1423.

Svarstad, B. L., Bultman, D. C., & Mount, J. K. (2004). Patient counseling provided in community pharmacies: Effects of state regulation, pharmacist age, and busyness. *J Am Pharm Assoc, 44*(1): 22-29.

Takiya, L. N., Peterson, A. M., & Finley, R. S. (2004). Meta-analysis of interventions for medication adherence to antihypertensives. *Ann Pharmacother, 38*(10): 1617-1624.

Trostle, J. A. (1997). Patient compliance as an ideology. In Gochman, D. S. (Ed.), *Handbook of health behavior research II: Provider determinants* (pp. 109-122). New York: Plenum.

Trostle, J. A., Hauser, W. A., & Susser, I. S. (1983). The logic of noncompliance: Management of epilepsy from the patient's point of view. *Cult Med Psychiatry, 7:* 35-56.

Vik, S. A., Maxwell, C. J., & Hogan, D. B. (2004). Measurement, correlates, and health outcomes of medication adherence among seniors. *Ann Pharmacother, 38*(2): 303-312.

Wahl, C., Gregoire, J. P., Teo, K., Beaulieu, M., Labelle, S., Leduc. B., Cochrane, B., Lapointe, L., & Montague, T. (2005). Concordance, compliance and adherence in healthcare: Closing gaps and improving outcomes. *Healthc Q, 8*(1): 65-70.

Weiden, P. J., Kozma, C., Grogg, A., & Locklear, J. (2004). Partial compliance and risk of rehospitalization among California Medicaid patients with schizophrenia. *Psychiatr Serv, 55*(8): 886-891.

WHO. *Adherence to long-term therapies-evidence for action.* 2003. Available at: http://www.who.int/chronic_conditions/en/adherence_report.pdf. Accessed May, 2005.

Williams, L. K., Pladevall, M., Xi, H., Peterson, E. L., Joseph, C., Lafata, J. E., Ownby, D. R., & Johnson, C. C. (2004). Relationship between adherence to inhaled corticosteroids and poor outcomes among adults with asthma. *Allergy Clin Immunol, 114*(6): 1288-1293.

Wilson J., Axelsen, K., & Tang, S. (2005). Medicaid prescription drug access restrictions: Exploring the effect on patient persistence with hypertension medications. *Am J Manag Care,* Spec No: SP27-34.

Ziegelstein, R. C., Fauerbach, J. A., Stevens, S. S., Romanelli, J., Richter, D. P., & Bush, D. E. (2000). Patients with depression are less likely to follow recommendations to reduce cardiac risk during recovery from a myocardial infarction. *Arch Intern Med, 160:* 1818-1823.

Chapter 4

The Costs of Noncompliance

INTRODUCTION

Compliance is often thought of (as it should be) in terms of the-rapeutic success or failure. If patients can reach a certain level of compliance an improvement in symptom may occur, a lessening of disease morbidity might be seen, or there might be a possibility of achieving a total cure. Conversely, if there is noncompliance, predictable contin-uation of symptoms, worsening of disease, or worse yet death may occur depending upon the condition being considered. Problems with patient compliance are similar across diseases, regimens, and age groups (Dunbar-Jacob et al., 2000). Compliance is an equal opportu-nity problem.

Patient noncompliance can have significant economic ramifica-tions as well. What is known is that a small segment of our population (5 percent) accounts for 49 percent of all overall cost expenditures in the U.S. health care system (Conwell & Cohen, 2005). Some of this expenditure of funds is no doubt attributable to noncompliance with drug therapies and ramifications related to patient behaviors. What follows is what we do know about the economic consequences of noncompliance.

The ramifications of noncompliance and commentary on this are not new; the issue of noncompliance with therapies, including vacci-nations, such as small pox, date back centuries (Nelson & Rogers, 1992). A decade ago, Feldman and DeTullio (1994) noted in general terms the economic ramifications of noncompliance, and more speci-fically, Scott (1996) indicated that the costs of compliance amounted to billions annually and would be a target of health plans so as to re-

Patient Compliance with Medications: Issues and Opportunities
© 2007 by The Haworth Press, Inc. All rights reserved.
doi:10.1300/5365_04

duce downstream costs. The economics of noncompliance upon downstream health care expenditures are significant predictors of health care costs (Cleemput & Kesteloot, 2002).

Johnson and Bootman (1995) were the first to more quantitatively target costs of drug-related morbidity, pegging the costs at $76.6 billion per year, some of which were attributable to noncompliance. Costs of drugs lead to a certain amount of noncompliance (Kennedy, Coyne, & Sclar, 2004), which no doubt can lead to further costs as a result of the initial lack of compliance. Kennedy and colleagues (2004) note that a significant number of adults with disabilities are noncompliant, and half of these individuals report on negative health consequences as a result. Millar and colleagues (2003) suggest that installment dispensing (trial therapy for a short duration) may be a method to enhance compliance and reduce the impact of noncompliance, both therapeutically and economically. Lack of health literacy leading to noncompliance and increased (Olshaker et al., 1999) costs have also been noted in the literature (Feifer, 2003). For example, an Australian study (Dartnell et al., 1996) notes that one-fourth of drug-related admissions to a hospital were attributed to noncompliance on the part of patients.

Admissions to emergency departments have also been tied to patient noncompliance. Dennehy and colleagues (1996) determined in one large-scale study that 58 percent of drug-related illnesses were tied to patient noncompliance across many disease states. Medication cost related noncompliance was also noted as a reason for emergency room visits in another study (Olshaker et al., 1999). In this study noncompliance with albuterol and phenytoin were the two most commonly identified offending drugs.

Twenty years ago, Pauly (1986) noted that physicians need to adopt a cost-conscious approach to treating hypertension. Prescribing without making an effort to understand the relationship between noncompliance and the high cost of drugs leads to noncompliance. Assuring patient compliance is a shared responsibility, and factors related to cost of therapy need to be considered in the selection of treatments and regimens (Claydon & Efron, 1994). Delgado (2000) notes that cost is one of several factors leading to noncompliance; collaborative treatment environments are a significantly important method of dealing with patient compliance as a shared responsibility.

Several diseases or specific conditions have been identified as severely impacted by patient noncompliance. In numerous cases, the cost of drug therapy is the main reason for noncompliance. Asthma, cardiovascular and cerebrovascular disease, diabetes, miscellaneous infections, and seizures are specific diseases that have been identified. And the elderly, antipsychotic medications, and transplantation are special classes of drugs or patient demographic groups singled out for economic problems due to noncompliance.

ASTHMA

The high price of asthma medications has been noted as but one reason for patient noncompliance (Petkova & Dimitrova, 2002). Elsewhere, Rubin (2004) discusses noncompliance due to cost of medications as an etiologic factor when patients describe the lack of effectiveness of their medications. Noncompliance with treatment guidelines leading to inappropriate use of beta agonist inhalers in four large HMOs (N = 673,000) led to an increase of three times the expenditures for patients following guidelines and using inhaled anti-inflammatory agents (Stempel, Durcannin-Robbins, Murphy, & Miller, 1996). Thus noncompliance can occur with both patients and providers and can lead to increased costs that include major expenditures of hospital and institutional services as opposed to less costly ambulatory services in treating asthma.

CARDIOVASCULAR AND CEREBROVASCULAR DISEASE

A cap on the number of prescriptions in a state Medicaid program that could be filled on a monthly basis was shown to lead to noncompliance with varying medications, notably drugs for cardiac conditions (Schulz, Lingle, Chubon, & Coster-Schulz, 1995). In private pay patients, noncompliance due to the costs of cardiac medications can also lead to extra expenditures (Hussey, Hardin, & Blanchette, 2002). Physicians notoriously underestimate patient compliance with cardiac medications (Dusing, Weisser, Mengden, & Vetter, 1998).

Prescribers need to ascertain the potential of the patients compliance with costly cardiac medications. When considering the high rate of noncompliance with antihypertensive regimens, cost is an important factor leading to patient noncompliance (Clark, 1991). In an examination of compliance barriers in hypertensive patients, noncompliance was found to be higher with higher drug treatment costs by various researchers (Bailey, Lee, Somes, & Graham, 1996; Richardson, Simons-Morton, & Annegers, 1993; Zyczynski & Coyne, 2000). Rizzo and Simons (1997) found that noncompliance with varying hypertensive therapies invariably led to higher ultimate health care costs (hospitalizations, further morbidity, etc.). Mar and Rodriguez-Artajelo (2001) note that hypertensive patients are heterogeneous and so are the options for treatments. They suggest matching therapeutic goals with achievable patient and drug therapy characteristics, including cost, so as to gain the best opportunities for success. Neal (1989) suggested years ago that treatment decisions take into consideration quality of life impacts, benefits of treatment, and costs associated with treatment relative to the therapeutic efficacy of the drugs in question. Finally, Neutel (1999) suggests low-dose combination therapies taken once daily to enhance compliance and lower costs at the same time, as opposed to using monotherapies at high doses that may also be expensive.

Noncompliance with prescribed therapy places the 500,000 stroke patients (per year in the United States) at risk for additional strokes or temporary ischemic attacks (TIAs) (Pecini, 1995; Schmidt & Jue, 1994).

DIABETES

In 1985, Fishbein found that 44 to 54 percent of a population of Rhode Island diabetics accessed through a statewide registry were noncompliant with diet and/or drug therapy. Hospitalizations and readmissions were more common in the noncompliant group. In a previously discussed study, Schulz et al. (1995) found that in a Medicaid population of diabetics, patients did not fill prescriptions due to the cost of drugs and an out-of-pocket outlay requirement. In a recently published research article from the antihypertensive and lipid-lowering treatment to prevent heart attack trial (ALLHAT), diuretics alone were shown to work as well as angiotension-converting enzyme inhibitors (ACE-inhibitors) and calcium channel blockers in protecting against heart attack and improving survival and to offer more protection against congestive heart failure (Whelton et al., 2005). This is important for several reasons, one of which is that in addition to these findings, the price of diuretics is less than that of agents in the other classes of drugs as well.

INFECTIOUS DISEASE

Pichichero (2000) speaks to the issue of noncompliance with antibiotics for respiratory infections. The points brought up include suggestions that both overprescribing of antibiotics and subsequent noncompliance is costly, both economically (costs of therapy leading to noncompliance, and lack of compliance leading to bacterial resistance and subsequent additional costs; and therapeutically (superinfections due to use over and above necessary lengths). Spiritus (2000) notes again, with respiratory tract infections, that lack of compliance with antibiotics leads to additional costs and suggests that once-daily regimens may make compliance more attainable. Ballow (1995) as well notes that the indirect and direct costs of noncompliance are so significant that once-daily regimens, although appearing to be more expensive, may in fact be less costly in the long run. Rosenberg and Waugh (1995) noted similar concerns and ramifications pertaining to drug treatment for pelvic inflammatory disease.

Concerning drug treatment for AIDS, the high cost of oral medications leads to noncompliance and lack of control of symptoms and the further progression of the disease (Skeel & Self, 1998). HIV patients are at risk for noncompliance (Morse et al., 1991). In addition, HIV patients with depression suffer many more symptoms due to noncompliance (Harel et al., 1996; Puzantian & Dopheide, 1995).

Noncompliance with tuberculosis chemotherapy has hastened the presence of drug-resistant strains (Bloch, Simone, McCray, & Castro, 1996; Davidson & Le, 1992; Houston & Fanning, 1994). Noncompliance and HIV infection are special issues in the treatment of tuberculosis (Humma, 1996). Pediatric patients with tuberculosis are affected as well (Starke, 1996). Overuse and misuse of antibiotics has led to the emergence of resistant nosocomial bacteria. With the ramifications of noncompliance with some tuberculosis medications being so significant, more invasive methods of ensuring compliance have been suggested. Uplekar and colleagues (1999) and Osman (1994) discuss the pros and cons of observational compliance for tuberculosis.

SEIZURES

Snodgrass and colleagues (2001) found that noncompliance with seizure medications in pediatric populations (as measured by anticonvulsant blood levels) was significantly correlated with socioeconomic variables, including family income. Uninsured patients were more at risk for noncompliance due to the inability to purchase medications. Noncompliance with antiepileptic therapies places patients at risk for increased seizure activity (Chadwick, 1995).

Specific subgroups of patients or patients taking certain drugs with varying classes have compliance-related economic ramifications worth mentioning as well. These include the elderly, transplantation patients, and patients taking antipsychotic agents.

THE ELDERLY

Compliance in elderly populations is a complex issue (Herrier, 1995). In a qualitative analysis of elderly drug-taking, Thompson (1996) suggested numerous opportunities to promote the quality use of medicine including the following:

- Accurate and specific labeling of prescription medications,
- Providing adequate drug information, and
- Monitoring for adverse affects.

These suggestions have been seconded by Corby and O'Donovan (1995).

One thing is clear—the elderly are no more noncompliant than other age groups because of their age (Lorence & Branthwaite, 1993).

However, many attributes predispose the elderly to noncompliance, including the following:

- social isolation,
- chronic diseases,
- multiple drug regimens,
- complex drug regimens, and
- severity of disease.

However, even these factors may not apply to all groups of elderly patients (Coons et al., 1994). Alzheimer's disease is a devastating disease with many effects, including a worsening of problems with noncompliance (Philpot & Puranik, 1995). Community-based compliance education has been suggested by Buerger (1995), as the potential of influencing elderly noncompliance. Specific places the elderly find themselves in, such as hospices (Burch & Hunter, 1996), are ideal sites to examine the specific medication needs of the elderly.

The results of elderly noncompliance are devastating. Bero and colleagues (1991) found that 35 percent of elderly patients are readmitted to hospitals with drug-related problems within six months of initial discharge. Drug-related factors were a major reason, rather than a contributing reason for 50 percent of the readmissions.

Underuse, overuse, misuse, and borrowing behavior are common factors to consider with elderly drug-taking. Salzman (1995) noted that underuse in the elderly can approach 40 percent, and finances are a major reason. The impact of Medicare Part D upon the financing of necessary prescriptions for the elderly remains to be seen. Crealey and colleagues (2003) suggest a standardized assessment of outcomes of drug use in pharmaceutical care programs with a focus on the elderly. Klein and colleagues (2004) suggest monitoring how payment changes affect seniors at risk for noncompliance. Some of the elderly cannot afford the cost of medications regardless of price. Skipping doses of drugs to economize is a deliberate attempt by some seniors (Steinman, Sands, & Covinsky, 2001). Wright (1988) suggests that due to the high cost of hypertensive medications and requirements by the elderly, the traditional stepped-care approach to treating hypertension may be impractical because patients cannot afford to try multiple drugs required in stepped therapy that can be expensive. Noncompliance with antidepressant medications can impact the 10 percent of the elderly estimated to suffer from depression. Compliance with selective serotonin reuptake inhibitors (SSRIs) may be more cost-effective than conventional treatments (Hughes, Morris, & McGuire, 1997), but the additional costs of these newer agents, which in turn may lead to noncompliance, may diminish their advantages. Elderly noncompliance can have significant downstream cost attributes. Malhotra and colleagues (2001) noted that a third of elderly emergency room visits were due to noncompliant patient behaviors.

With the elderly, it is not age per se that makes the issue of noncompliance so crucial; it is the multiple morbidities and extent of such that becomes critical with seniors. Complex drug therapies also serve to fester noncompliant behavior. Noncompliance knows respects no age; however, the characteristics of the elderly place them at risk.

ANTIPSYCHOTIC THERAPY

Chronic mental health patients exhibit poor noncompliance (Kelly & Scott, 1990). In a study examining the revolving door admission–readmission phenomenon in a sample of chronically ill mental patients, alcohol and drug problems and noncompliance were identified as major factors related to mental facility readmissions (Haywood et al., 1995). Antipsychotic medications are affected by noncompliance, affect additional expenditure if not complied with, and also impact issues of right to refuse treatment for personal reasons. Noncompliance with antipsychotic medications has been estimated to be 60 percent after one year, and only 25 percent after two years (Perkins, 1999). Approximately one-half of schizophrenic patients are compliant, and noncompliance leads to relapse, hospitalization, poor outcomes, and obvious economic costs (Bebbington, 1995; Perkins, 2002). Relapse rates of schizophrenics due to noncompliance have been estimated to cost billions annually (Weiden & Olfson, 1995). In the United Kingdom, a recent estimate suggested that noncompliance with antipsychotics increases system costs by a factor of three (Knapp, King, Pugner, & Lapuerta, 2004). Brown and colleagues (1999) have noted that atypical antipsychotics have higher acquisition costs and better compliance options than conventional therapies. However, older conventional neuroleptics may be the first-choice therapies strictly due to cost characteristics. Elsewhere, Coley et al. (1999) found that the high-acquisition costs of respiridone are not offset by a reduction in relapse tares when compared with conventional antipsychotics. To more fully assess the long-term consequences, both therapeutic and economic, with noncompliance with schizophrenic medications, Thieda and colleagues (2003) suggest longitudinal assessments as a better tool than short-term evaluations.

Regarding treatment of depression, compliance with selective serotonin reuptake inhibitors (SSRIs) has been found to be better than compliance with tricyclic antidepressants (TCAs), but Anderson and Tomenson (1995) caution against overestimatation of the benefits of SSRIs. But even with the newer agents, noncompliance is still a problem (Delgado, 2000). Rates of noncompliance with bipolar treatment is also a factor in additional, more costly expenditures (Durrenberger, Rogers, Walker, & de Leon, 1999).

TRANSPLANTATION PHARMACOTHERAPY

Financial restrictions impact compliance behaviors in transplantation recipients (Paris, Dunham, Sebastian, Jacobs, & Nour, 1999; Swanson, Hull, Bartus, & Schweizer, 1992). Economically, the resultant costs of patient noncompliance with medications after transplantation versus the costs of renal dialysis have been debated, as not being much more expensive after noncompliance (Cleemput, Kesteloot, Vanrenterghem, & De Geest, 2004). The authors conclude that even with noncompliance, renal transplantation is more cost-effective than traditional dialysis therapy. However, this noncompliance can lead to adverse treatment outcomes that entail further costly interventions (Loghman-Adham, 2003). From a societal standpoint, should society "pay" (by paying for additional costly interventions), when transplant recipients do not "pay" according to expectations (Minuth, 1992)?

Noncompliance with other medications, such as oral contraceptives, will lead to obvious ramifications. These include a potential unplanned pregnancy and the associated costs of childbirth and beyond. Specific examples were not given for the health condition of pregnancy, but the significance of such noncompliance goes without saying.

In summary, patients who are noncompliant extract more resources from the health care system and cause more morbidity and monetary expenditures through their noncompliance. This noncompliance by many differing types of patients is caused by many factors; one of the main variables is the cost of medications and the subsequent inability of patients to pay, eventually leading to noncompliance.

REFERENCES

Anderson, I. M. & Tomenson, B. M. (1995). Treatment discontinuation with selective serotonin reuptake inhibitors compared with tricyclic antidepressants: A meta-analysis. *Bmj, 310*(6992): 1433-1438.

Bailey, J. E., Lee, M. D., Somes, G. W., & Graham, R. L. (1996). Risk factors for antihypertensive medication refill failure by patients under Medicaid managed care. *Clin Ther, 18*(6): 1252-1262.

Ballow, C. H. (1995). Cost considerations in oral antibiotic therapy. *Adv Ther, 12*(4): 199-206.

Bebbington, P. E. (1995). The content and context of compliance. *Int Clin Psychopharmacol, 9*(5): 41-50.

Bero, L. A., Lipton, H. L., & Bird, J. A. (1991). Characterization of geriatric drug-related hospital readmissions. *Med-Care, 29*(October): 989-1003.

Bloch, A. B., Simone, P. M., McCray, E., & Castro, K. G. (1996). Preventing multidrug-resistance tuberculosis. *JAMA, 275*(February 14): 487-489.

Brown, C. S., Markowitz, J. S., Moore, T. R., & Parker, N. G. (1999). Atypical antipsychotics: Part II: Adverse effects, drug interactions, and costs. *Ann Pharmacother, 33*(2): 210-217.

Buerger, D. (1995). How to start a community-based education program. *Consult-Pharm, 10*(August): 852, 849.

Burch, P. L., & Hunter, K. A. (1996). Pharmaceutical care applied to the hospice setting; a cancer pain model. *Hosp J, 11*(3): 56-59.

Chadwick, D. (1995). Do anticonvulsants alter the natural course of epilepsy? Case for early treatment is not established. *Br-Med-J, 310*(January 21): 177-178.

Clark, L. T. (1991). Improving compliance and increasing control of hypertension: Needs of special hypertensive populations. *Am Heart J, 121*(2 Pt 2): 664-669.

Claydon, B. E., & Efron, N. (1994). Non-compliance in general health care. *Ophthalmic Physiol Opt, 14*(3): 257-264.

Cleemput, I., & Kesteloot, K. (2002). Economic implications of non-compliance in health care. *Lancet, 359*(9324): 2129-2130.

Cleemput, I., Kesteloot, K., Vanrenterghem, Y., & De Geest, S. (2004). The economic implications of non-adherence after renal transplantation. *Pharmacoecon, 22*(18): 1217-1234.

Coley, K. C., Carter, C. S. , DaPos, S. V., Maxwell, R., Wilson, J. W., & Branch, R. A. (1999). Effectiveness of antipsychotic therapy in a naturalistic setting: A comparison between risperidone, perphenazine, and haloperidol. *J Clin Psychiatry, 60*(12): 850-856.

Conwell, L. J., & Cohen, J. W. *Characteristics of Persons with High Medical Expenditures in the U.S. Civilian Noninstitutionalized Population,* 2002. Statistical Brief #73. March 2005. Agency for Healthcare Research and Quality, Rockville, MD. http://www.meps.ahrq.gov/papers/st73/stat73.pdf.

Coons, S. J., Sheahan, S. L., Martin, S. S., Hendricks, J., Robbins, C. A., & Johnson, J. A. (1994). Predictors of medication noncompliance in a sample of older adults. *Clin Ther, 16*(1): 110-117.

Corby, D., & O'-Donovan, D. (1995) Can the community pharmacist improve geriatric compliance? *Ir Pharm J, 73*(March): 74, 76-77, 79, 82.

Crealey, G. E., Sturgess, I. K., McElnay, J. C., & Hughes, C. M. (2003). Pharmaceutical care programmes for the elderly: Economic issues. *Pharmacoecon, 21*(7): 455-465.

Dartnell, J. G., Anderson, R. P., Chohan, V., Galbraith, K. J., Lyon, M. E., Nestor, P. J., et al. (1996). Hospitalisation for adverse events related to drug therapy: Incidence, avoidability and costs. *Med J Aust, 164*(11): 659-662.

Davidson, P. T., & Le, H. Q. (1992). Drug treatment of tuberculosis. *Drugs, 43:* 651-673.

Delgado, P. L. (2000). Approaches to the enhancement of patient adherence to antidepressant medication treatment. *J Clin Psychiatry, 61*(2): 6-9.

Dennehy, C. E., Kishi, D. T., & Louie, C. (1996). Drug-related illness in emergency department patients. *Am J Health Syst Pharm, 53*(12): 1422-1426.

Dunbar-Jacob, J., Erlen, J. A., Schlenk, E. A., Ryan, C. M., Sereika, S. M., & Doswell, W. M. (2000). Adherence in chronic disease. *Annu Rev Nurs Res, 18:* 48-90.

Durrenberger, S., Rogers, T., Walker, R., & de Leon, J. (1999). Economic grand rounds: The high costs of care for four patients with mania who were not compliant with treatment. *Psychiatr Serv, 50*(12): 1539-1542.

Dusing, R., Weisser, B., Mengden, T., & Vetter, H. (1998). Changes in antihypertensive therapy—the role of adverse effects and compliance. *Blood Press, 7*(5-6): 313-315.

Feifer, R. (2003). How a few simple words improve patients' health. *Manag Care Q, 11*(2): 29-31.

Feldman, J. A., & DeTullio, P. L. (1994). Medication noncompliance: An issue to consider in the drug selection process. *Hosp Formul, 29*(3): 204-211.

Fishbein, H. A. (1985). Precipitants of hospitalization in insulin-dependent diabetes mellitus (IDDM): A statewide perspective. *Diabetes Care, 8*(1): 61-64.

Harel Z., Biro, F. M., Kollar, L. M., & Rauh, J. L. . (1996). Adolescents' reasons for and experience after discontinuation of the long-acting contraceptives Depo-Provera and Norplant. *J Adolesc Health, 19*(2): 118-123.

Haywood, T. W., Kravitz, H. M., Grossman, L. S., Cavanaugh, J. L. Jr, Davis, J. M., & Lewis, D. A. (1995). Predicting the "revolving door" phenomenon among patients with schizophrenic schizoaffective, and affective disorders. *Am J Psychiatry, 152*(6): 856-861.

Herrier, R. N. (1995). Medication compliance in the elderly. *J Pharm Pract, 8*(October): 232-244.

Houston, S., & Fanning, A. (1994). Current and potential treatment of tuberculosis. *Drugs, 48*(November): 689-708.

Hughes, D., Morris, S., & McGuire, A. (1997). The cost of depression in the elderly. Effects of drug therapy. *Drugs Aging, 10*(1): 59-68.

Humma, L. M. (1996). Prevention and treatment of drug-resistant tuberculosis. *Am J Health Syst Pharm, 53*(October 1); 2291-2298, 2335-2337.

Hussey, L. C., Hardin, S., & Blanchette, C. (2002). Outpatient costs of medications for patients with chronic heart failure. *Am J Crit Care, 11*(5): 474-478.

Johnson, J. A., & Bootman, J. L. (1995). Drug-related morbidity and mortality. A cost-of-illness model. *Arch Intern Med, 155*(18): 1949-1956.

Kelly, G. R., & Scott, J. E. (1990). Medication compliance and health education among outpatients with chronic mental disorders. *Medical Care, 28:* 1181-1197.

Kennedy, J., Coyne, J., & Sclar, D. (2004). Drug affordability and prescription noncompliance in the United States: 1997-2002. *Clin Ther, 26*(4): 607-614.

Kennedy, J., & Erb, C. (2002). Prescription noncompliance due to cost among adults with disabilities in the United States. *Am J Public Health, 92*(7): 1120-1124.

Klein, D., Turvey, C., & Wallace, R. (2004). Elders who delay medication because of cost: Health insurance, demographic, health, and financial correlates. *Gerontologist, 44*(6): 779-787.

Knapp, M., King, D., Pugner, K., & Lapuerta, P. (2004). Non-adherence to antipsychotic medication regimens: Associations with resource use and costs. *Br J Psychiatry, 184:* 509-516.

Loghman-Adham, M. (2003). Medication noncompliance in patients with chronic disease: Issues in dialysis and renal transplantation. *Am J Manag Care, 9*(2): 155-171.

Lorence, L., & Branthwaite, A. (1993). Are older adults less compliant with prescribed medication than younger adults? *Br J Clin Psych, 32:* 485-492.

Malhotra, S., Karan, R. S., Pahndi, P., & Jain, S. et al. (2001). Drug related medical emergencies in the elderly: Role of adverse drug reactions and non-compliance. *Postgrad Med J, 77*(913): 703-707.

Mar, J., & Rodriguez-Artalejo, F. (2001). Which is more important for the efficiency of hypertension treatment: Hypertension stage, type of drug or therapeutic compliance? *J Hypertens, 19*(1): 149-155.

Millar, J., MacKinnon, W., Struther, M., & Vance, C. (2003). A pilot study to investigate the use of installment dispensing as a method of reducing drug wastage owing to adverse drug reactions. *Br J Gen Pract, 53*(492): 550-552.

Minuth, A. N. (1992). The economic load of the noncompliant patient: Must society pay for the shrew? *Artif Organs, 16*(1): 98-101.

Morse, E. V., Simon, P. M., Coburn, M., Hyslop, N., Greenspan, D., & Balson, P. M. (1991). Determinance of subject compliance within an experimental anti-HIV drug protocol. *Soc Sci Med, 32:* 1161-1167.

Neal, W. W. (1989). Reducing costs and improving compliance. *Am J Cardiol, 63*(4): 17B-20B.

Nelson, M. C., & Rogers, J. (1992). The right to die? Anti-vaccination activity and the 1874 smallpox epidemic in Stockholm. *Soc Hist Med, 5*(3): 369-388.

Neutel, J. M. (1999). Low-dose antihypertensive combination therapy: Its rationale and role in cardiovascular risk management. *Am J Hypertens, 12*(8 Pt 2): 73S-79S.

Olshaker, J. S., Barish, R. A., Naradzay, J. F., Jerrard, D. A., Safir, E., & Campbell, L. (1999). Prescription noncompliance: Contribution to emergency department visits and cost. *J Emerg Med, 17*(5): 909-912.

Osman, H. (1994). Tuberculosis in AIDS patients: An ethical dilemma for discharge planning. *Disch Plann Update, 14*(5): 1, 3-7.

Paris, W., Dunham, S., Sebastian, A., Jacobs, B., & Nour, C. (1999). Medication nonadherence and its relation to financial restriction. *J Transpl Coord, 9*(3): 149-152.

Pauly, M. V. (1986). The changing health care environment. *Am J Med, 81*(6C): 3-8.

Pecini, M. (1995). Pharmacist-managed ticlopidine clinic. *Am J Health Syst Pharm, 52*(September 15): 2030-2031.

Perkins, D. O. (1999). Adherence to antipsychotic medications. *J Clin Psychiatry, 60* (21): 25-30.

Perkins, D. O. (2002). Predictors of noncompliance in patients with schizophrenia. *J Clin Psychiatry, 63*(12): 1121-1128.

Petkova, V., & Dimitrova, Z. (2002). Asthma, drug medication and noncompliance. *Boll Chim Farm, 141*(5): 355-356.

Philpot, M., & Puranik, A. (1995). Psychotropic drugs and community care. *New-Ethicals, 32*(October): 23-24, 26-28.

Pichichero, M. E. (2000). Short course antibiotic therapy for respiratory infections: A review of the evidence. *Pediatr Infect Dis J, 19*(9): 929-937.

Puzantian, T., & Dopheide, J. A. (1995). Major depression in patients with HIV infection and AIDS. *Calif Pharm, 42*(February): 27-32.

Richardson, M. A., Simons-Morton, B., & Annegers, A. F. (1993). Effect of perceived barriers on compliance with antihypertensive medication. *Health Educ Q, 20*(4): 489-503.

Rizzo, J. A., & Simons, W. R. (1997). Variations in compliance among hypertensive patients by drug class: Implications for health care costs. *Clin Ther, 19*(6): 1446-1457; discussion 1424-1425.

Rosenberg, M. J., & Waugh, M. S. (1995). Consequences of incomplete antibacterial treatment for chlamydial pelvic inflammatory disease. *Drugs, 49*(2): 504-505.

Rubin, B. K. (2004). What does it mean when a patient says, "my asthma medication is not working?" *Chest, 126*(3): 972-981.

Salzman, C. (1995). Medication compliance in the elderly. *J Clin Psychiatry, 56* (1): 18-22; discussion 23.

Schmidt, B. A., & Jue, S. G. (1994). Detecting potential medication adherence problems in stroke patients: Implications for pharmacists' interventions. *ASHP-Annual-Meeting, 51*(June); P-86(D).

Schulz, R. M., Lingle, E. W., Chubon, S., & Coster-Schulz, M. A. (1995). Drug use behavior under the constraints of a Medicaid prescription cap. *Clin Ther, 17*(2): 330-340.

Scott, L. (1996). Providers push for remedies to costly drug noncompliance. *Mod Healthc, 26*(16): 44-46, 48, 50.

Skeel, J. D., & Self, D. J. (1988). AIDS and the allocation of limited resources: Admissions to intensive care units. *J Crit Care, 3*(3): 195-198.

Snodgrass, S. R., Vedanarayanan, V. V., Parker, C., & Ruth, B. (2001). Pediatric patients with undetectable anticonvulsant blood levels: Comparison with compliant patients. *J Child Neurol, 16*(3): 164-168.

Spiritus, E. (2000). Antibiotic usage for respiratory tract infections in an era of rising resistance and increased cost pressure. *Am J Manag Care, 6*(23): S1216-S21.

Starke, J. R. (1996). Tuberculosis in children. *Prim Care, 23*(4): 861-881.

Steinman, M. A., Sands, L. P., & Covinsky, K. (2001). Self-restriction of medications due to cost in seniors without prescription coverage. *J Gen Intern Med, 16*(12): 793-799.

Stempel, D. A., Durcannin-Robbins, J. F., Murphy, D. M ., & Miller, S. B. (1996). Drug utilization evaluation identifies costs associated with high use of beta-adrenergic agonists. *Ann Allergy Asthma Immunol, 76*(2): 153-158.

Swanson, M., Hull, D. Bartus, S., & Schweizer, R. (1992). Economic impact of non-compliance in kidney transplant recipients. *Transplant Proc, 24*(6): 2722.

Thieda, P., Beard, S., Richter, A., & Kane. J. (2003). An economic review of compliance with medication therapy in the treatment of schizophrenia. *Psychiatr Serv, 54*(4): 508-516.

Thompson S. (1996). Opinions and prescription medication use practices among the non-institutionalised elderly. Doctoral Thesis, Victorian College of Pharmacy, Monash University, Melbourne, Victoria, Australia.

Uplekar, M., Walley, J., & Newell, J. (1999). Directly observed treatment for tuberculosis. *Lancet, 353*(9147): 145; author reply 147-148.

Weiden, P. J., & Olfson, M. (1995). Cost of relapse in schizophrenia. *Schizophr Bull, 21*(3): 419-429.

Whelton, Paul K., Barzilay, J., Cushman, W. C., Davis, B., Ilamathi, E., & Kostis, J. (2005). Clinical outcomes in antihypertensive treatment of Type 2 diabetes, impaired fasting glucose concentration, and normoglycemia: Antihypertensive and lipid-lowering treatment to prevent heart attack trial (ALLHAT). *Arch Intern Med, 165:* 1401-1409.

Wright, J. T., Jr. (1988). Geriatric hypertension therapy: A guide to cost-effectiveness. *Geriatrics, 43*(8): 55-62.

Zyczynski, T. M., & Coyne, K. S. (2000). Hypertension and current issues in compliance and patient outcomes. *Curr Hypertens Rep, 2*(6): 510-514.

Chapter 5

Definitions and Measurement of Compliance

The definition of compliance is important for both patients and providers. It is not fair to label patients in one manner and not let them know how to improve or change their categorization. It is probably not fair to categorize people at all. Labels do not help patients, and, more than likely, are damaging to patient–provider interactions. It is useful for providers to understand the past compliance behavior of patients.

Providers need to understand patient compliance behaviors. Interventions cannot be tailored to meet patient therapeutic needs if patient drug-taking behavior is unclear. Conversely, if patient drug-taking patterns are discernable, it is possible to help patients take medications as they should through varying types of compliance interventions. These interventions may include patient counseling (verbal or written), specialized packaging (unit of use, unit dose, blister packs, specialized containers, and/or packaging of medications to be taken at the same time in the same unit of use containers), varying refill reminders (letters mailed, e-mailed, telephone calls, etc.), or perhaps other types of specialized contacts.

Obviously, if we cannot measure how patients are taking medications, it is not possible to formulate specialized aids to help patients take medications. Measurement of compliance can vary as we shall see from mildly invasive to very invasive. Patients and providers can be asked whether compliance there is compliance, and the veracity of each of the responses is subject to verification. Blood levels can be measured, therapeutic outcomes can be measured, and indirect methods of estimating compliance (side effects, certain outcomes of

Patient Compliance with Medications: Issues and Opportunities
© 2007 by The Haworth Press, Inc. All rights reserved.
doi:10.1300/5365_05

drug use examined) can all be undertaken with varying assurances of accuracy.

Definitions and measurement are tenuous unless something can be accomplished by ensuring patient compliance, or better compliance. For this, patients must be seen as partners in the process and not as subjects to be manipulated or harshly evaluated for errors in their medication compliance. Nothing can turn a patient from cooperative to leery more quickly than "catching them doing something wrong" as opposed to assessing nonjudgmentally why there is noncompliance behavior.

Compliance estimates on behalf of patients should be considered for inclusion in "vital signs" sections of medical records, electronic, or otherwise. These compliance estimates can be viewed as equally important as the other crucial measures that are included in assessing patients. Blood pressure measurements are isolated determinations if assessing the adherence to treatment regimens to treat the hypertension are also not concomitantly assessed and recorded. Pulse values for a congestive heart failure patient are of little use if compliance with treatments is not also assessed at the same time. One cannot hide values for weight, height, temperature, blood pressure, and/or pulse readings when having vital signs evaluated and recorded. In the same vein, patients need to feel nonthreatened to have compliance estimates gleaned and recorded in patient medical records. This may take multiple entries for multiple drugs consumed, and be time consuming. But, it would appear to be a very good use of time and energy. Assuming patients are compliant when they actually are not, and, subsequently, not providing additional, individualized compliance aids or further pharmacotherapy that might be easier complied with is more time consuming and vastly more costly for all involved.

DEFINITIONS OF COMPLIANCE

The definitions used to categorize patients as compliant or noncompliant have varied tremendously. This variance in defining compliance has been suggested to be problematic (Dunbar-Jacobs, Dwyer, & Dunning, 1991). Compliance is certainly not an "either or" patient behavior; thus the definitions of compliance behavior must be varied to reflect eclectic patient behaviors. Please see Exhibit 5.1 for several definitions of varying types of compliance. Patients can certainly progress from one of these types of compliance to another. Please see Figure 5.1 for a depiction of a continuum of compliance activities (Fincham, 1995; Fincham, 2005; Fincham & Wertheimer, 1988). Figure 5.2 presents an updated depiction, which indicates that the complexity of compliance is much more fluid and can detail several points of shifting from one type of compliance behavior to another.

Patients who are taking multiple therapies may actually be in several of these categories at the same time with several types of medications they may be consuming. Certainly these depictions would have to be repeated for each of the varying drugs that a patient may be taking. It is also possible that patients may be varyingly compliant with several medications at the same time. The depiction of the spheres of compliance activity in the figure should definitely be considered to be fluid and subject to changes in behavior based on the myriad factors that have been related to compliance behavior by differing patients consuming differing drug therapies at any juncture in their disease treatments.

Noncompliance is not a new construct; it has been referred to for long periods of time in many written forms (Sbarbaro & Steiner,

EXHIBIT 5.1. Definitions of varying forms of compliance.

Initial compliance. The patient receives a written prescription, and transfers it to a pharmacy; or has the prescription phoned to a pharmacy, but does not wait or return to pick up the filled prescription. Patients who do not present written prescriptions for filling could be included in this group.

Partial compliance. The process of taking a prescribed and dispensed medication at a level less than the prescriber or dispenser intended.

Compliance. The process of complying with a prescribed and dispensed regimen precisely as the prescriber or dispenser intend. Compliance may also refer to a therapeutic endpoint, such as normotension for hypertensive patients.

Hypercompliance. The situation whereby a patient takes a prescribed and dispensed medication at a level over and above the recommended and intended dosing interval.

Initial Compliance → Partial Compliance → Compliance → Hypercompliance

FIGURE 5.1. The compliance continuum.

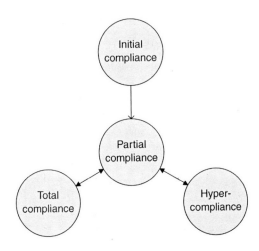

FIGURE 5.2. The interrelationship of various types of compliance.

1991). Mention of the problem of noncompliance has been made numerous times in the medical, pharmacy, and nursing literature. The topic has also been noted in the lay press (Kjellgren, Ahlner, & Saljo, 1991), where noncompliance has been described as risky.

Fawcett (1995) suggest adherence as the word to use when examining patient drug-taking behaviors:

> Instead of "compliance," it has been suggested that the term adherence be used, which puts more of a burden on the clinician to form a therapeutic alliance with the patient, which thereby increases behavioral compliance and possibly enhances the therapeutic effect of the medication administered. (p. 5)

The consequences and ramifications of patient noncompliance with medication regimens pervade all aspects of the delivery of health care. Noncompliance has the potential to be deleterious to pharmaceutical manufacturers, prescribers, dispensers, patients, and society as a whole.

While not all factors affecting patient noncompliance have been quantified, a growing body of research and knowledge has been accumulating to shed light on the noncompliance problem. Potential impacts upon medication nonadherence have been formulated, instituted, and evaluated. Despite the steady increase of advances regarding the knowledge of noncompliance, much work remains to be done.

Drug manufacturers, patients, and providers have come to the realization that the problem of medication noncompliance does not rest with one segment of the health care system. Just as the problem pervades all aspects of health care delivery, the responsibility for finding a solution to the understanding and reversal of patient noncompliance (where it is appropriate to do so) must also be shared. Pharmaceutical manufacturers must strive to formulate pharmaceuticals that help to facilitate medication consumption. Manufacturers must follow up the prescribing and dispensing of pharmaceuticals to ascertain if in fact the formulation, packaging, or dosage form design of a product enhances patient compliance with that compound. Physicians most certainly must share in the responsibility for patient compliance. Post-prescribing follow-up of patients should be undertaken to ascertain proper drug selection for individual patient needs, both in the therapeutic- and compliance-related sense of medication requirements. Certainly the writing of a prescription must not signal the end of physician involvement in medication compliance considerations of patients. Patients must be made responsibe, and be given input for, the medication regimens they are required to take. The patient could be the individual most responsible for the final compliance decision. If aspects of a medication regimen are unacceptable, patients must inform physicians and pharmacists of their wishes, desires, problems, or concerns.

Before patients reach the stage of being noncompliant with drug therapies, they initially enter the health care system at varying entry points. They may see a physician, a pharmacist, or perhaps both. They may also bypass the professionals entirely and self-medicate with drugs obtained from others. Before examining self-medication or noncompliance any further, the reasons for patients entering the health care system must be examined. Patients enter the health care system with varying intents and a multiplicity of purposes. Pharmacists may see patients at the beginning, midpoint, or at the end of their entry into the health system. Pharmacists should seek a firm understanding of why patients enter the formal health care system and what they seek to obtain.

NONCOMPLIANCE: NEGATIVE CONNOTATIONS

Regardless of the setting studied or the terms used to describe noncompliance, the connotations are certainly negative. The cooperative patient is stated to be compliant, undemanding, or accepting. The uncooperative patient is referred to as difficult, recalcitrant, unreasonable, or demanding (Powers & Ford, 1976). Assigning such a negatively charged label to a patient does no good if there is not a corresponding effort to understand actions, either by the patient or health professionals, which may lead a patient into noncompliance.

MEASUREMENT OF COMPLIANCE

Recently, novel methods of compliance measurement have been designed and evaluated. Researchers, not surprisingly, struggle to agree on whether there is a gold standard measure of compliance. Wood and Gray (2000) suggest: "There has not been a 'gold standard' identified for measuring compliance, therefore it is difficult to compare results due to differences in operational definitions" (p. 1).

Elsewhere, Hill and colleagues (2003) write:

> Although there are gold standards for adherence measurement, such as directly observed therapy, these measurements are most frequently used to classify respondents as adherers or nonadherers based on whether they take a certain percentage of their medication. Such a categorization is simplistic and does not reflect the complexity of adherence patterns. (p. 520)

Nevins (2005) writes concerning pediatric noncompliance:

> The problem of compliance or adherence with medical advice is complex in every aspect. Frequently compliance definitions vary, measurements are not well quantified, interventions are uncontrolled or not fully elaborated. (p. 847)

So what is one to do? Assuming that there is not one agreed-upon standard, creativity is called for. Because no "gold standard" for compliance measurement exists, innovative technologies have been applied with positive results (Von Renteln Kruse, 1997). One such method, continuous dosage monitoring, records the time of bottle opening. In one study, this electronic assessment of compliance provided evidence of seizure-related noncompliance not evidenced by history, drug serum concentrations, or total pill counts.

As a further layer of complexity in measurement of compliance, it is necessary to combine medication compliance with compliance with nutritional requirements in order to evaluate compliance, for example, with hypertensive patients (The Treatment of Mild Hypertension Research Group, 1991). Compliance with one aspect of care and noncompliance with other aspects can lead to outcomes that do make sense if only considering one of the compliance behaviors. So the hypertensive patient who complies with medications at a level of 95 percent, but does not follow dietary prescriptions (low sodium diet, etc.) and remains hypertensive, may lead caregivers to assume that the drug just did not work. In another example, treatment for alcohol addiction can be evaluated not only by drugs consumed (naltrexone or disulfiram) but also by blood alcohol determinations (Anton et al., 1999). In the same light, treatments for smoking cessation, other than nicotine, can be assessed by also examining cotinine levels (Woodward & Tunstall-Pedoe, 1992).

METHODS TO DETECT COMPLIANCE

Several methods have been utilized to detect compliance. These methods include interrogation of the patient, tablet estimates,[1] markers,[2] drug detection in serum, or failure to dispense (Von Renteln Kruse, 1997). Of these five methods, the failure to dispense method is the most accurate method of measuring noncompliance. Claxton and colleagues (2001) write:

> Previous reviews of the literature on medication compliance have confirmed the inverse relationship between number of daily doses and rate of compliance. However, compliance in most of these studies was based on patient self-report, blood-level moni-

toring, prescription refills, or pill count data, none of which are as accurate as electronic monitoring (EM). (p. 1298)

In an evaluation of the various methods available for the detection of compliance, Rapoff and Christophersen (1982) have rank ordered the measures of compliance according to their objectivity. Their rating of compliance measures listed from most to least objective is as follows:

- Assay (blood, urine, feces, saliva)
- Observational methods
- Pill counts
- Treatment outcome
- Physician estimates (overestimate compliance)
- Patient reports

Rapoff and Christophersen (1982) concluded their assessment of compliance measures by stating, "One reason for the failure of investigators to specify the definition of acceptable compliance is the lack of a clearly objective or universal method for classifying patients as compliant or noncompliant" (p. 92). Researchers also try a combination of measures, such as pill counts and blood-level determinations (Beck et al., 1992). Lim (1992) suggests several problems with reliance on blood-level determinations of compliance: ". . . problems of false-positivity, false-negativity, and bias that arise because of experimental errors in the drug assays, pharmacokinetic variations of the drug, and differential dosing levels" (p. 620).

Elixhauser and colleagues (1990), when evaluating compliance with lithium, used self-report, lithium levels, appointment keeping, and medication refill records. Patient reports of compliance behavior can be evaluated by self-reports of patients (Krapek et al., 2004); the Compliance Scale asks patients whether they ever forget to take medication, whether they are careless about taking medication, and whether they ever stop taking medication (Morisky, Green, & Levine, 1986).

Missed doses do not automatically equate with therapeutic failures, in hypertensive patients. Ongtengco and colleagues (2002), when purposefully examining the results of two missed doses, found that patients could still control blood pressure with these two omitted doses.

Rudd (1998), when examining the current situation with hypertensive therapy and compliance, notes: "Based on this analysis, current levels of hypertension detection, treatment, and control remain suboptimal" (p. 960).

Basically, because not one or several measures are unquestionably reliable, researchers use several measures to try to evaluate compliance behavior.

Weiden and colleagues (2004) used four differing compliance definitions in a study of schizophrenia patients:

- gaps in medication therapy (e.g., days without therapy),
- medication consistency (e.g., taking at the appropriate time),
- medication persistence (e.g., use over time), and
- medication possession ratio (e.g., days of therapy remaining based on doses remaining in the patients' possession).

PHYSICIANS' ESTIMATES OF THEIR PATIENTS' COMPLIANCE

Several compliance investigators have researched the ability of physicians to estimate their patients' compliance. Some have questioned whether a physician even considers the possibility of noncompliance in a patient population (Stoeckle, 1987). It may be wise to exercise caution in considering physicians and their ability to make judgments of their patients' compliance behavior.

Finally, Hayes and Lucas (1999) have questioned physician compliance. These researchers noted that only 59 percent of eligible patients receive angiotensin converting enzyme (ACE) inhibitors and only two-thirds receive thrombolysis or angioplasty.

CAN PHYSICIANS BE NONCOMPLIANT?

Certainly physicians taking medications can be just as susceptible to noncompliance as any patient taking medications. Whether physicians are personally more compliant or noncompliant than others is an empirical question, but is really not worth researching. Patients are patients regardless of professional or other denotations that might otherwise separate subpopulations of patients and their compliance behaviors. Noncompliance knows no class or hierarchical boundaries separating patients.

Perhaps a more useful interpretation of this question might be how compliant are physicians in their drug-prescribing activities? Schoni and colleagues (1995) examined pediatric patient compliance in light of appropriateness of physician-prescribing compliance and concluded that inappropriate physician-prescribing behavior dramatically affects patient compliance. Compliance has been viewed in such a paternalistic light that perhaps the tables should be turned and an examination of prescribers and dispensers should be closely studied. There are gold standard treatments for varying conditions, and in some cases, physicians ignore these and prescribe inappropriate therapies. Physicians also prescribe therapies and multiple regimens without much, if any, consideration of how patients may struggle to comply with the agents. Bergman and Wilholm (1981) point out that inappropriate medication doses, or administration times, which ignore normalized pharmacokinetic parameters, can easily lead patients into noncompliant behaviors.

In summary, the definitions of compliance can help patients understand where they are with medication taking, and where they need to be to obtain optimal therapy outcomes. Measurement of compliance is a mechanism to help patients and providers understand the level of appropriate drug use by patients.

NOTES

1. This could also include capsules or liquid: the balance of the remaining drug is compared with what was dispensed to determine whether the appropriate amount was taken for a specified period of time.

2. When either the patient's urine or feces is examined, it is possible to see the marker, usually a chemical, in the material excreted.

REFERENCES

Anton, R. F., Moak, D. H., Waid, L.R., Latham, P. K., Malcolm, R. J., & James, K., & Dias, J. D. (1999). Naltrexone and cognitive behavioral therapy for the treatment of outpatient alcoholics: Results of a placebo-controlled trial. *Am J Psychiatry, 156*(11): 1758-1764.

Beck, R. A., Mercado, D. L., Seguin, S. M., Andrade, W. P., & Cushner, H. M. (1992). Cardiovascular effects of pseudoephedrine in medically controlled hypertensive patients. *Arch Intern Med, 152*(6): 1242-1245.

Bergman, U., & Wilholm, B. E. (1981). Drug-related problems causing admission to a medical clinic. *Eur J Clin Pharmacol, 20*(3): 193-200.

Claxton, A. J., Cramer, J., & Pierce, C. (2001). A systematic review of the associations between dose regimens and medication compliance. *Clin Ther, 23*(8): 1296-1310.

Dunbar-Jacobs, J., Dwyer, K., & Dunning, E. J. (1991). Compliance with antihypertensive regimen: A review of research in the 1980s. *Ann BehavMed, 13*(1): 31-39.

Elixhauser, A., Eisen, S. A., Romeis, J. C., & Homan, S. M. (1990). The effects of monitoring and feedback on compliance. *Med Care, 28*(10): 882-893.

Fawcett, J. (1995). Compliance: Definitions and key issues. *J Clin Psychiatry, 56*(Suppl 1): 4-8; discussion 9-10.

Fincham, J. E. (1995). Medication compliance and the elderly. *J. Pharmacoepidem, 4*(2): 7-14.

Fincham, J. E. (2005). *Taking your medicine: A guide to medication regimens and compliance for patients and caregivers.* Binghamton, NY: The Haworth Press.

Fincham, J. E., & Wertheimer, A. I. (1988). Elderly patient initial noncompliance: The drugs and the reasons. *J Ger Drug Ther, 2*(4): 53-62.

Hayes, G., & Lucas, B. (1999). Tools for improving compliance. *Pat Care, 33*(15): 15-16.

Hill, Z., Kendall, C., & Fernandez, M. (2003). Patterns of adherence to antiretrovirals: Why adherence has no simple measure. *AIDS Pat Care STDS, 17*(10): 519-525.

Kjellgren, K. I., Ahlner, J., & Saljo, R. (1995). Taking hypertensive medication—controlling or co-operating with patients? *Int J Cardiol, 47*(3): 257-268.

Krapek, K., King, K., Warren, S. S., George, K. G., Caputo, D. A., Mihelich, K., et al. (2004). Medication adherence and associated hemoglobin A1c in type 2 diabetes. *Ann Pharmacother, 38*(9): 1357-1362.

Lim, L. L. (1992). Estimating compliance to study medication from serum drug levels: Application to an AIDS clinical trial of zidovudine. *Biometrics, 48*(2): 619-630.

Morisky, D. E, Green, L. W., & Levine, M. D. (1986). Concurrent and predictive validity of a self-reported measure of medication adherence. *Medical Care, 24:* 67-74.

Nevins, T. E. (2005). Why do they do that? The compliance conundrum. *Pediatr Nephrol, 20*(7): 845-848.

Ongtengco, I., Morales, D., Wilkinson, R., & Singh, S. (2002). Persistence of the antihypertensive efficacy of amlodipine and nifedipine GITS after two "missed doses": A randomised, double-blind comparative trial in Asian patients. *J Hum Hypertens, 16*(11): 805-813.

Powers, M. J., & Ford, L. C. (1976). The best kept secret: Consumer power and nursing potential. In Lasagna, L, (Ed.), *Patient compliance* (pp. 131-139). Mt. Kisco, NY: Futura Publishing Co.

Rapoff, M. A., & Christophersen, E. R. (1982). Compliance of pediatric patients. In Stuart, R. B., (Ed.), *Adherence, compliance and generalization in behavioral medicine* (pp. 245-259). New York: Brunner-Mazel.

Rudd, P. (1998). Compliance with antihypertensive therapy: Raising the bar of expectations. *Am J Manag Care, 4*(7): 957-966.

Sbarbaro, J. A., & Steiner, J. F. (1991). Noncompliance with medications: Vintage wine in new (pill) bottles. *Annals of Allergy, 66:* 273-275.

Schoni, M. H., Horak, E., & Nikolaizik, W. (1995). Compliance with therapy in children with respiratory diseases. *Eur J Pediatr, 154*(9 Suppl 4): S77-81.

Stoeckle, J. D. (1987). *Encounters between patients and doctors: An anthology.* Cambridge, MA, US: The MIT Press.

The Treatment of Mild Hypertension Research Group. (1991). The treatment of mild hypertension study. A randomized, placebo-controlled trial of a nutritional-hygienic regimen along with various drug monotherapies. The Treatment of Mild Hypertension Research Group. *Arch Intern Med, 151*(7): 1413-1423.

Von Renteln Kruse, W. (1997). Recording methods in regard to patient compliance in medical practice: Clinical trials and consequences. *PZ-Prisma, 4*(October): 189-194.

Weiden, P. J., Kozma, C., Grogg, A., & Locklear, J. (2004). Partial compliance and risk of rehospitalization among California Medicaid patients with schizophrenia. *Psychiatr Serv, 55*(8): 886-891.

Wood, W., & Gray, J. (2000). An integrative review of patient medication compliance from 1990-1998. *Online J Knowl Synth Nurs, 7:* 1.

Woodward, M., & Tunstall-Pedoe, H. (1992). Biochemical evidence of persistent heavy smoking after a coronary diagnosis despite self-reported reduction: Analysis from the Scottish Heart Health Study. *Eur Heart J, 13*(2): 160-165.

Chapter 6

Models to Evaluate
Patient Compliance

Christopher Cook

Noncompliance of prescribed medication regimens continues to be a tremendous burden on the health care system and represents a modifiable behavior that can be addressed to improve treatment outcomes. Identification of the factors that underlie medication noncompliance and interventions to improve medication compliance has become the focus of a great deal of research in the health care field. Unfortunately, much of this research has been atheoretical in nature and not grounded in established behavioral theory. The purpose of this chapter is to provide an overview of the theoretical frameworks that have been examined in the literature to further our understanding of the medication compliance behavior. Research in this area has been primarily motivated by the desire to reduce the prevalence of noncompliance of therapy, improve patient outcomes to treatment and so effect improvements in the health and lives of our individual patients as well as in the overall health of the population.

Before discussing individual models, a brief introduction is needed of what psychology has found out about changing health behavior. In general, the study of health behavior is based upon two primary assumptions—that a significant amount of morbidity and mortality is caused by particular behavior patterns and that these behavioral patterns can be modified (Stroebe & Stroebe, 1995). Within behaviors, epidemiological studies have demonstrated that considerable variation

Patient Compliance with Medications: Issues and Opportunities
© 2007 by The Haworth Press, Inc. All rights reserved.
doi:10.1300/5365_06

exists between individuals who will perform a given desired behavior. So, in trying to identify the underlying factors for this variation in medication compliance behavior, a large number of specific variables have been presented in the literature (Fincham & Wertheimer, 1985). However, all these individual specific variables can be placed in one of two broad categories: factors either intrinsic or extrinsic to the individual (Conner & Norman, 1996a). Intrinsic factors include factors specific to the individual such as sociodemographics, personality, social support, and cognitions. Extrinsic factors are considerations affecting behavior in the individual's environment but are not specific to the individual. Health policy falls into this category. These extrinsic factors have been subclassified as either incentive structures (e.g., multitiered medication insurance copayment, reduced copayment for use for in-network physicians) or legal restrictions (e.g., access to legend drugs only by a prescribing authority, public smoking bans) (Conner & Norman 1996b). The intrinsic factors have received predominant attention from psychologists with the cognitive factors such as beliefs, attitudes, and knowledge being focused upon as the most important determinants to behavioral change. Models that utilize these cognitive factors to produce behavioral change are referred to as social cognitive models. It is this group of behavioral models that encompass the largest percentage of theory-based research in the medication compliance literature and it is these models that will primarily be the focus of this chapter.

Social cognitive models are concerned with how individuals make sense of various social situations. The general approach focuses on how an individual's thoughts are modifiable processes that occur between the stimuli and the response in a real-world situation (Fiske & Taylor, 1991). For medication compliance behavior, the self-regulation processes are of primary concern and bring about the desired behavioral change. Self-regulation processes can be defined as "mental and behavioral processes by which people enact their self-conceptions, revise their behavior, or alter their environment so as to bring about outcomes in it in line with their self-perceptions and personal goals" (Fiske & Taylor, 1991, p. 450). Self-regulation encourages the setting of goals, cognitive preparations, and continuous evaluation of progress and goal monitoring. In medication compliance behavior, the practitioner seeks to empower patients to achieve their treatment goals related to maintaining or improving their health.

Another characteristic of social cognitive models is that each model provides a list of important targets or determinants from which interventions can be designed to focus upon in order to change behavior successfully. An underlying principle among the models is that behavioral actions are based on rational decision-making, which is a result of deliberate, systematic, review of the available information. While the criteria involved may be subjective for each individual, every action is assumed to be based on an assessment of the information. The individual then makes a cost-benefit type analysis of the likely outcomes of the available response options. It is assumed that individuals generally attempt to maximize utility and so prefer behaviors that are associated with the greatest expected benefit to personal outcomes. The social cognitive models discussed in this chapter include the health belief model, theory of reasoned action, the theory of planned behavior, the social cognitive theory, and the transtheoretical model. In addition, several of the more prominent behavioral models in the psychology of behavioral change are briefly covered at the end of the chapter.

HEALTH BELIEF MODEL

The Health Belief Model (HBM) is one of the oldest and most widely used social cognitive models in health psychology. The model was developed in the early 1950s by a group of social psychologists, at the United States Public Health Service, who were developing models that would identify appropriate targets for health education programs. Originally, the model was utilized to study which people would adopt preventative health behaviors or use health services (Hochbaum, 1958; Rosenstock, 1966). Later, the model was applied to patients' responses to symptoms and to following prescribed medical regimens (Becker, 1974; Kirscht, 1974).

Components of the HBM are derived from various psychological and behavioral models which hypothesize that behavior depends upon two main variables: (1) the value placed by an individual on a particular goal and (2) the individual's estimate of the likelihood that a given action will achieve that goal (Maiman and Becker, 1974). When these variables are conceptualized in context with health behavior, they become (1) the desire to avoid illness or get well, and (2) the belief that a specific health action will prevent or cure illness (Clark and Becker, 1998). The HBM integrates six distinct constructs dealing with the individual's perception as well as other nonspecific variables that may modify the individual's decision toward the health action in question (see Figure 6.1). Within the HBM, sociodemographic factors operate to influence these determinants of behavioral intention.

The HBM measures threat perception, or an individual's desire to avoid or recover from an illness, through the following variables: perceived susceptibility and perceived severity. The perceived susceptibility construct refers to one's subjective belief of the risk of contracting a condition. The perceived severity construct measures the feelings concerning the seriousness of contracting an illness (or leaving an illness untreated). The severity construct includes both the evaluations of medical and clinical consequences as well as possible social consequences.

The HBM measures behavioral evaluation, or the individual's belief of the consequences of a specific health action, through perceived benefits and perceived barriers. The perceived benefits construct ex-

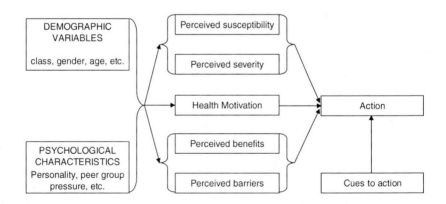

FIGURE 6.1. The Health Belief Model. (*Source:* Sheeran, P. & Abraham, C. [1996]. The Health Belief Model. In M. Conner & P. Norman (Eds.), *Predicting health behaviour: Research and practice with social cognition models* (p. 26). Philadelphia, PA: Open University Press. Reprinted with permission of McGraw-Hill.

amines the beliefs regarding the feasibility and effectiveness of the various actions available in reducing the threat of disease. The perceived barriers construct assesses the potentially negative aspects of a particular health action that may impede the undertaking of a recommended behavior. A type of cost-benefit analysis is then performed by the individual through the weighing of the benefits versus the costs of the health action. In addition, the cues to action construct was proposed to account for diverse triggers to health behaviors when appropriate beliefs are held. Perception of symptoms, social influence, and health education campaigns are examples of the types of cues that could influence an individual's health behavior. Last, health motivation or readiness to be concerned about health matters was added in later versions of the model (Becker, Maiman, Kirscht, Haefner, & Drachman, 1977).

Becker, as early as 1976, summarizes the use of the HBM in medication compliance behavior in a review article as follows: "Most studies have produced internally consistent findings in the predicted direction; taken together they yield relatively strong support for the conceptual model of the compliance behavior" (Becker, 1976, p. 135). Since this review, numerous studies in medication compliance have utilized the HBM. While the studies mentioned here do not form an exhaustive list from the literature, they are intended to provide a sample of the work in this area. Fincham and Wertheimer utilized components of the HBM to investigate the attitudes of initial drug-defaulters versus those of initial compliers and found a 20 percent explanation of variance (Fincham & Wertheimer, 1985). A number of studies have examined psychiatric populations with the model reported to explain anywhere from 0 to 43 percent of the variance (Adams & Scott, 2000; Budd, Hughes, & Smith, 1996; Connelly, Davenport, & Nurnberger, 1982; Kelly, Mamon, & Scott, 1987; Pan & Tantam, 1989). The inconsistent findings in this population could be a result of various methods used in the studies or reflective of the inherent difficulty in measuring the medication compliance behavior. Application in other therapies has been examined and range widely from asthma (Putman, 2002) to bipolar disorders (Scott, 2002) to diabetes (Alogna, 1980; Brownlee-Duffeck, Peterson, Eidsen, & Delamater, 1987; Cerkoney & Hart, 1980; Chao, 2004) to malaria prophylaxis (Abraham, Clift, & Grabowski, 1999). Additional support for the constructs of the HBM can be found in its combined use with other behavioral theories as will be discussed later in this chapter.

THEORY OF REASONED ACTION

The Theory of Reasoned Action (TRA) is the development from Ajzen and Fishbein's (1980) beliefs that the cause of volitional behaviors is the result of one's intention to perform a behavior (Ajzen & Fishbein, 1980). The theory is a product of Fishbein's early work on how attitude might cause behavior. Fishbein based this early work on the value-expectancy framework by Peak and thus it utilizes the same underlying principles as other value-expectancy models (Peak, 1955). Even though the model was not developed with health behaviors in mind, it has been adapted to include a number of health-related behaviors.

The model states that one's behavioral intentions are a reflection of one's attitudes about the action, one's beliefs about the perceptions others will have to that action (subjective norms), and how important the individual's desire is to please or submit to the wishes of others (see Figure 6.2).

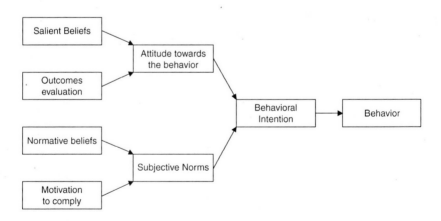

FIGURE 6.2. Theory of reasoned action. (*Source:* Reprinted from *Social Science and Medicine, 27*(3), Reid, L. D., & Christensen, D. B., *A psychosocial perspective in the explanation of patients' drug-taking behavior* [1988]: 277-285. With permission from Elsevier.)

The TRA, therefore, establishes a link between behavioral intention and the actual behavior. It also specifies the relationships and causal processes among the determinants. While the TRA is similar to the HBM in that the sociodemographic factors operate only to influence the determinants of the behavioral intention, the inclusion of subjective norms as a determinant has been found to add a strong cultural component to the prediction of behavior. One limitation to emphasize is that the TRA applies only to volitional behaviors or behaviors of choice. Thus, behaviors requiring skills, resources, or opportunities in order to be performed will likely be poorly predicted by this model (Terry, Gallois, & McCamish, 1993).

Several articles in the literature have addressed the use of the TRA in medication compliance positively. Reid and colleagues examined the applicability of the TRA in explaining medication compliance intentions among 300 males taking antihypyertensive medications (Ried, Oleen, Martinson, & Pluhar, 1985). A regression analysis found the independent variables of the model predicted 35 percent of the variance. In addition, a path analysis showed that attitudes and subjective norms produced the greatest direct impact upon intention to take the medication as prescribed. The variables of susceptibility and physicians' normative expectations also were found to be significant in medication-taking intentions. A later study by Reid and Christensen (1988) examined the applicability of the HBM and TRA models in predicting drug-taking compliance behavior among thirty-eight female patients with uncomplicated urinary tract infections (Ried & Christensen, 1988). The study found that the HBM variables of barriers and benefits were significant in medication compliance and that a stepwise regression model using the HBM variables was able to explain 10 percent of the variance. The significant TRA variables of belief strength, outcome evaluation, and behavioral intentions were then added to the model using a hierarchical regression procedure and were found to contribute an additional 19 percent explanation of variance to the model for a total of 29 percent variance explanation using the combined models. Additional supporting studies include medication compliance in disulfiram treatments (Brubaker, Prue, & Rychtarik, 1987), lithium regimens (Cochran and Gitlin, 1988), and rheumatoid arthritis therapy (Lorish, Richards, & Brown, 1990).

One article by Miller, Wikoff, and Hiatt (1992) found negative path analysis results for the TRA structure in medication compliance (Miller et al., 1992). Fifty-six newly diagnosed hypertensive patients completed the variable measures of attitude, perceived beliefs of others, and motivation to comply six months after beginning a therapy. The path analysis found the TRA model sufficient to describe prescribed treatment for diet, smoking, activity, and stress, but was insufficient in its explanation of medication compliance. For medication compliance, attitude and motivation to comply were found to directly influence regimen compliance rather than directly influencing intention which, in turn, should influence regimen compliance directly as described by the model. In conclusion, the TRA has been utilized in a number of studies addressing medication compliance with the majority of studies providing support for the model.

THEORY OF PLANNED BEHAVIOR

An extension of the TRA has been developed by Ajzen called the Theory of Planned Behavior (TPB) (Ajzen, 1985). Expansion of the model was designed to increase the application of the TRA to include nonvolitional behaviors. Modification of the model was accomplished by giving specific consideration regarding the determinant perception of control over performance. Thus, the theory states that the performance of a behavior is a function of the intentions to engage in a behavior and the control the person has over that behavior (see Figure 6.3). By this addition, the application of the theory was increased from beyond easily performed, volitional, behaviors to be applicable in more complex goals and behaviors (Conner & Norman, 1996a). Hence, the TPB may be the more appropriate of Ajzen's two models when the probability of success and actual control over performance of a behavior is less than perfect as in medication compliance behavior.

The intention to perform a behavior is theorized to be determined by the strength of three constructs; attitude toward the behavior, subjective norms, and perceived control. Attitude toward the behavior is the overall evaluation of the individual toward the behavior. The determinants of the attitude component are the individual's perceived

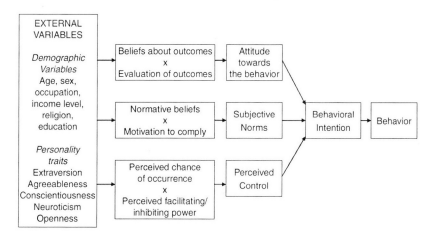

FIGURE 6.3. Theory of planned behavior. (*Source:* Adapted from Conner, M., & Sparks, P. [1996]. The theory of planned behavior and health behaviors. In Conner, M., & Norman, P. (Eds.), *Predicting health behavior: Research and practice with social cognitive models* (p. 128). Philadelphia: Open University Press. Reprinted with permission).

consequences of successfully completing or failing to complete the behavior in question and the individual's evaluation of these consequences. The subjective norms component is the same as in the TRA, and is a function of normative beliefs, or the person's beliefs about the opinion that significant others will approve or disapprove of the behavior. The last component, perceived control over the behavior, may include both internal control factors (skills, knowledge, ability, emotions, will power) as well as external control factors (opportunity, dependence on others, money, barriers). This determinant is similar to the self-efficacy construct described by Bandura (1977), and which forms the key determinant in the social cognitive theory that is discussed later in the chapter. People who perceive themselves as having the resources to accomplish a task and the opportunity to perform the behavior will have a higher level of perceived control. Each of these three determinants—attitude, social norms, and perceived control—contributes to the overall intention of the individual to perform the behavior. Thus, the more positive the attitude, the greater the acceptance within social norms, and the greater the perceived control over the personal and external factors that may interfere with the behavior, the greater the likelihood that the behavior will be performed (Ajzen, 1985).

The theory of planned behavior has been utilized in several studies of medication compliance behavior. Conner, Black, and Stratton examined the TPB in a psychiatric population and found that 38.1 percent of medication compliance variance was explained by intentions and perceived behavioral control. In addition, 65 percent of the construct intentions to comply with the drug regimen was explained through attitudes, subjective norms, and perceived behavioral control (Conner et al., 1998). In a study by Costa in 1999, subjective norms, attitudes, and perceived behavioral control constructs explained 88 percent of the variance in the construct intensions to manage the therapeutic regimen in patients with heart failure. Intentions were then able to explain 27 percent of the variance in the reported health behaviors of these patients (Costa, 1999).

Several researchers have combined various elements of the HBM and the theory of planned behavior to explain medication compliance. Abraham, Clift, and Grabowski tested a combined model in malaria prophylaxis adherence and reported approximately 50 percent explanation of variance among mefloquine users and a 40 percent explanation among chloroquine and proguanil users (Abraham et al., 1999). Putman tested a combined model in rural Appalachian adults with asthma. Health beliefs explained 26.4 percent of the variance in compliance behaviors, while attitude toward the illness and behavioral intentions to comply explained 22.7 percent and 15.8 percent, respectively. Putnam emphasized that health beliefs and behavioral intention to comply explained more in medication compliance than any one variable independently (Putman, 2002). Thus, while moderate success has been found using the TPB determinants alone, one may want to consider a combination with HBM constructs in an effort to increase the explanation of medication compliance behavior.

SOCIAL COGNITIVE THEORY

In 1977, the concept of self-efficacy was introduced by Albert Bandura and it is this construct that would later form the key determinant of the social cognitive theory (Bandura, 1977). In addition to self-efficacy, the social cognitive theory also specifies knowledge, outcome expectations, goals, perceived facilitators, and perceived impediments as the determinants of the model (Figure 6.4). Knowledge of health risks and benefits of different health behaviors forms the overall precondition needed for change. Without an individual having the knowledge and understanding of the need for a behavioral change, there will not be a sincere attempt by the individual to adopt healthier behaviors. If the individual does not comprehend that the risks of a disease state may be reduced or controlled through compliance of a medication regimen, it is unlikely that the individual will ever adhere to a prescribed course of therapy. So, knowledge of the health behavior in question, and the behavioral change required, is necessary to adequately create and assess the other determinants of self-efficacy, outcomes expectations, goals, and underlying socio-structural factors.

Bandura describes behavioral change as a function of an individual's expectations about the outcomes that will result from a particular behavior and the expectations the individual has in his/her own ability to accomplish the behavior or task. Thus, a distinction is made in Bandura's model between outcomes expectations and efficacy expectations. Outcomes expectations focus on the results or consequences if the behavior is performed whereas efficacy expectations focus on one's belief in their ability to perform the behavior. This distinction is made because even when an individual believes a certain change will enhance or improve their life, if that individual does not

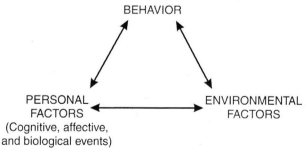

FIGURE 6.4. Social cognitive model. (*Source:* Adapted from Pajares, Frank (2002). *Overview of social cognitive theory and of self-efficacy.* Retreived August 8, 2006, from http://www.emory.edu/EDUCATION/mfp/eff.html.)

believe that he or she can execute the behavior required, the belief in needing to change alone will not influence the performance of the behavior. This thought process affects both the success of an individual to initiate a change as well as one's success in maintaining a change.

Perceived self-efficacy is the conviction that an individual can successfully execute a behavior needed to achieve a certain outcome. This fundamental construct has been found to determine whether a coping behavior will be initiated, how much effort an individual will put on a behavior and the ability of the individual to continue a behavior change in the face of adversity (Bandura, 1982; O'Leary, 1985; Velicer, DiClemente, Rossi, & Prochaska, 1990). Self-efficacy has become a focal determinant because of its direct effect on the health behavior and its influence on the other determinants (Bandura, 2004). The self-efficacy construct has gained such acceptance that its concept has been integrated into the HBM, the TPB, and the Transtheoretical model (TTM). An interesting point Bandura emphasizes is that efficacy expectations, or self-efficacy, is not a global trait that operates independently of contextual situations, but rather a confidence variable that may be strengthened or weakened depending on the circumstances involved (Bandura, 1986). In the context of medication compliance, a patient with diabetes may be confident of complying with a simple single daily dose regimen, but have low self-efficacy in their ability to comply with a complex multiple-injection sliding-scale insulin regimen based on carbohydrate counting. Therefore, Bandura emphasizes how perceptions influence behavior and that these perceptions are not necessarily in accordance with one's true capabilities.

Outcomes expectations can take several different forms: physical, social, and self-evaluative. Physical outcomes of a behavior include both the pleasurable events as well as the adverse consequence of a behavior. The social outcomes include the approval and disapproval that the behavior will produce from others. The self-evaluative outcomes consist of the positive and negative reactions one has to the behavior and the resulting health status. Individuals self-regulate their behaviors by performing what gives self-satisfaction and self-worth and by avoiding behaviors that create self-dissatisfaction.

Personal health goals help set the course for personal change and provide additional motivation and directional guidance. While the long-term goals may set the course, there are often too many competing influences in the short term for the long-term goals to control immediate behavior. Therefore, the setting of short-term attainable goals can often help provide assistance to individuals in achieving their long-term goals. By aligning the short-term goals with the long-term objectives, an individual can continue on the correct course without facing seemingly unobtainable endpoints that the long-term goals alone may represent.

Sociostructural factors consist of both the perceived facilitators as and the perceived impediments that may influence persons regarding the changes they seek. Some impediments are personal while other hindrances may be a result of the barriers inherent in the health system that deter the person from the health behavior. These barriers form an integral part of the self-efficacy assessment. If there were no barriers to overcome, then personal change would be easy. It is the perceived level of difficulty resulting from the barriers that influence the confidence an individual will have in being successful in the attempt at change.

The social cognitive model has been utilized to assess medication compliance in a number of chronic diseases. High self-efficacy has been associated with improved adherence in diabetes (Kavanagh, Gooley, & Wilson, 1993; McCaul, Glasgow, & Schafer, 1987; Senecal, Nouwen, & White, 2000), epilepsy (DiIorio, Hennessy, & Manteuffel, 1996), rheumatoid arthritis (Taal, Rasker, Seydel, & Wiegman, 1993), and HIV (Smith, Rublein, Marcus, Brock, & Chesney, 2003; Tuldra et al., 2000). Kavanagh, Gooley, and Wilson in a 1993 study of sixty-three patients with diabetes found that self-efficacy was a significant predictor of later compliance even after previous levels of adherence were taken into account. A regression model containing diabetes control, treatment type, and self-efficacy was able to explain over 50 percent of the variance in medication compliance (Kavanagh et al., 1993). Smith and colleagues in 2003 report that a self-management intervention based on the social cognitive theory is a potentially useful model for improving adherence to complex regimens such as HIV/ AIDS care (Smith et al., 2003). Resnick and colleagues have recently reported validation of two scales measuring self-efficacy and outcomes expectations in osteoporosis (Resnick, Wehren, & Orwig, 2003). In this study, the authors report that self-efficacy was able to explain 15 percent of medication adherence while outcome expectancy was able to account for an additional 2 percent of the variance in medication adherence. Lastly, Kalichman and colleagues have developed a visual analogue scale to assess medication adherence self-efficacy in low-literacy patients (Kalichman et al., 2005). Within this study, a possible solution to one of the difficulties of self-efficacy measures, highly positively skewed results, appears to have been presented. These initial studies provide support that self-efficacy and the social cognitive theory may provide a useful underpinning to medication compliance interventions.

TRANSTHEORETICAL MODEL

First introduced in 1982, the Transtheoretical Model (TTM) attempts to integrate previous psychotherapy research in a comprehensive approach to changing behavior. The TTM assumes that a model of behavioral change must be able to account for how people overcome problems on their own as well as how they change with the help of others. The model was developed by observing behavioral patterns of self-changers exhibited throughout their course of therapy. According to Prochaska et al. (1994), the model determinants and the interaction between the determinants ". . . hold for behaviors differing on such dimension as acquisition and cessation, addictive and non-addictive, frequent and infrequent, legal and illegal, public and private, and socially acceptable and less socially acceptable" (Prochaska et al., 1994, p. 39). Since the development of the model studying smoking cessation behavior, it has been applied in a number of health behaviors, including medication compliance.

The four main constructs of the TTM include the stages of change, processes of change, self-efficacy, and decisional balance. The most extensively studied of these four constructs has been the stages of change. The stages of change construct contain five dimensions that a person moves through during a behavioral change process: precontemplation, contemplation, preparation, action, and maintenance. It is the goal of the practitioner to assist the patient to advance through these stages until the behavioral change is complete. In medication compliance, the stages of change have been defined and are presented in Table 6.1.

TABLE 6.1. Stages of change construct definitions for medication compliance behavior.

Stage	Definitions
Precontemplation	The patient is not concerned about missed or off scheduled doses of his/her medication and has no intention of changing his/her medication taking behavior in the foreseeable future.
Contemplation	The patient is considering changing his/her medication taking behavior in the next few months and is somewhat concerned about missed or off scheduled doses.
Preparation	The patient is more concerned about missed or off scheduled doses and is intending to change his/her behavior in the near future (within the next thirty days).
Action	The patient has successfully started taking his/her medication as directed and has been doing so for less than six months.
Maintenance	The patient has continued to successfully take his/her medication for more than six months.

Precontemplation is the stage where the individual is unaware of the problem or for some reason has no consideration about changing the behavior. Overall, precontemplators tend to be defensive and distant about their own problems. They may begin a therapy to appease a concerned loved one but generally are at a higher risk of discontinuing a therapy and are likely to have feelings of being coerced by the efforts of others. Depending on the resistance of the person, the precontemplation stage may last from minutes to a lifetime.

Contemplation is defined by the individual's awareness that a personal problem exists but has yet to determine the need to make a behavioral change. The individual begins trying to understand the problem and its consequences. Often, during this time the individual actively seeks more information to assist in solving their problems. Persons in the contemplation stage tend to want to talk about the problem. Often one will seek reassurance that the problem can be understood and resolved. While the individual may appear anxious to learn about the problem, the move toward action may be slow until a full understanding is achieved. Therefore, the duration of this stage depends on the level of the problem, the amount of introspection of the person, as well as the amount of understanding that the individual requires before seeking treatment.

The next stage, preparation, is defined as when one is planning on changing behavior in the near future. The near future is a relative term depending on the characteristics of the behavior in question. In medication compliance, it has been defined as intending to change the behavior within the next thirty days. Often the person has established goals and made a commitment to change the behavior in question.

Preparation was not included in the original development of the TTM but has been added as a modification to the model. Previous research indicates that the preparation stage exists in many of the addictive behaviors where it appears that the lifestyle modification is significant. However, for medication compliance behavior, the preparation dimension has not been isolated (Cook & Perri, 2004; Johnson, Grimley, & Prochaska, 1998). This inability to detect the preparation stage in medication compliance behavior could be due to the relatively mild nature of the behavioral change in comparison to substance addictions. This relative mild change may create a preparation stage too short in duration to be easily captured in patient-reported measures. The question of the existence of the preparation stage in medication compliance has yet to be resolved in the literature.

The action stage represents the time where a person makes a conscious choice to change his or her behavior to resolve the problem. It is the most visible of the stages because the overt changes in behavior are recognizable to outsiders. While action is usually the shortest of the stages in duration of time, it is where the most progress is made. The action stage generally can last anywhere from one to six months depending on the individual and the behavior. One fallacious thinking of many people believe is that they only need will power to change their behavior. As a result, they often expend a tremendous amount of energy during this stage. Unfortunately, the enthusiasm for a behavioral change can only last so long. Due to this inability to maintain will power, many people will revert to the old behavior before they achieve the maintenance stage.

The maintenance stage is where the individual works to continue the successes of the action stage and to prevent a relapse. It is where the person continues to learn how to cope with the daily barriers or temptations that may interfere with the change in behavior. Fear of relapse is often present during this time resulting in persons often becoming rigid or structured in their everyday lives as though any change will result in a relapse. This fear of relapse frequently creates a long duration in the maintenance stage. Maintenance usually lasts at least six months, but it can last years or even a lifetime before an individual no longer fears a relapse.

If an individual does revert to the old behavior, relapse is the result. Most individuals slide back to the contemplation stage, but some will regress all the way back to precontemplation. The inclusion of the relapse concept creates a bidirectional feature of the stages of change construct, making it different from the typical stage model. In the majority of stage models, an individual progresses from one stage to another without revisiting a previous stage; however, the relapse concept is appropriate to describe a behavioral change process. Relapse can be very difficult to overcome because of the psychological damage caused to the one's self-esteem. Feelings of frustration, helplessness, and guilt often accompany the relapse and the person's sense of self-efficacy is shaken. These feelings can have serious repercussions on the efforts of the individual to try the behavior change again.

The conclusion to the stages of change construct is the termination of the behavioral change process. Termination occurs when the person no longer has any temptations to return to the previous behavior and no longer has to make efforts to keep from relapsing into the old behavior. Some patients will never experience this stage where the change is no longer a factor in their lives. The termination step is the exit through the revolving door of an unhealthy behavior.

The decisional balance construct is the weight an individual places on the perceived benefits (pros) against the perceived costs (cons) involved in adopting a new behavior. Research has demonstrated that decisional balance is a good predictor of successful change with a broad range of health-related behaviors (Prochaska et al., 1994). Prochaska and colleagues maintain that the pros and cons are excellent indicators of an individual's progress through the stages of change from precontemplation to contemplation to preparation (DiClemente et al., 1991; Prochaska, DiClemente, Velicer, Ginpil, & Norcross, 1985; Velicer, DiClemente, Prochaska, & Brandenburg, 1985). Prochaska has directed multiple longitudinal studies across various behaviors and has determined that the cons outweigh the pros during the precontemplation stage and that the pros outweigh the cons at the action and maintenance stages (Prochaska, Velicer, Guadagnoli, & Rossi, 1991; Prochaska et al., 1994). Depending on the behavior in question, the crossover appears to occur during the contemplation to preparation stages. Decisional balance appears most useful during the early stages in understanding and predicting transitions between precontemplation, contemplation, and preparation. During the later stages of action and maintenance, decisional balance appears less important as a predictor of progress.

The self-efficacy construct from Bandura's social cognitive theory comprises the third determinant in the TTM. Self-efficacy is defined as the conviction that one can successfully perform the behavior required to produce the desired outcome. Assessment of this construct often involves asking subjects to rate how tempted they would be to engage in a behavior, given a variety of situations, or how confident they are that they could avoid the behavior in a variety of situations. The self-efficacy construct has been found to increase almost linearly across the stages from precontemplation to maintenance (Grimley et al., 1996). In the precontemplation stage, self-efficacy is found to be at its lowest point and from there it begins to increase until it peaks in the action or maintenance stage. The self-efficacy construct is an important predictor of progress, especially during the later stages of action and maintenance.

Processes of change make up the final construct of the TTM. The processes of change construct is made up of a number of common strategies that have been consistently applied across various health behaviors. These strategies include consciousness raising, dramatic relief, self-reevaluation, environmental reevaluation, self-liberation, helping relationships, counterconditioning, reinforcement management, stimulus control, and social liberation. Use of these strategies varies across the stages of change with some of the strategies being of more use in certain stages. Dramatic relief has been useful for motivating individuals in the precontemplation stage to move into the contemplation stage. Self-reevaluation can be helpful to motivate persons from the contemplation stage onward toward action, while stimulus control can be particularly helpful to advance someone from action to maintenance (Rossi & Rossi, 1999).

Several articles have examined the application of the TTM in medication compliance. A 1998 study by Johnson, Grimley, and Prochaska evaluated the predictive ability of the constructs of the TTM against several static predictors in the area of medication compliance to oral contraceptives (Johnson et al., 1998). The population consisted of 306 contraceptive pill users in 2 clinic sites. The TTM constructs accounted for 42 and 44 percent of the variability in the two populations. The strongest to weakest of the TTM variables for predicting noncompliance appear to be stages of change, decisional balance, self-efficacy, and processes of change.

Willey and colleagues examined the use of the TTM in two populations: hypertensive patients and HIV-infected patients (Willey et al., 2000). Results from both diseases state populations supported the use of the model in medication compliance. In the HIV-infected population, a one-way ANOVA found that the stages of change construct showed significant differences in the level of medication compliance across stages ($F = 7.46$, $p < 0.001$) with similar support reported in the hypertensive population ($\chi^2 = 441.3$, $p = 0.001$).

This author has examined the utility of the TTM to explain medication compliance in five chronic disease states: diabetes, hypertension, hypercholesterolemia, hypothyroidism, and hormone replacement therapy (Cook & University of Georgia, 2002). Relationships between the TTM constructs were found to be consistent with those found in other health behaviors, validating the structure of the TTM in medication compliance behavior and the relationship between the various constructs of the model. Medication compliance increased across the stages of change construct ($F = 7.88$, $p = 0.0006$). Decisional balance ($F = 14.24$, $p < 0.0001$) and self-efficacy ($F = 5.73$, $p < 0.0039$) both significantly increased as patients progressed through the stages of change construct. Explanation of variance by the TTM constructs ranged from 9.6 to 41.1 percent depending on the measure of compliance used.

Additional studies have examined the application of the model in several differing disease states. Tutty, Simon, and Ludman tested a telephonic counseling intervention based on the TTM for patients with depression (Tutty, Simon, & Ludman, 2000). Patients in the counseling group showed significantly lower depressive symptoms at both the three-month and six-month timepoints as well as being twice as likely to adhere to the antidepressant medication. A study of HIV-positive males demonstrated the level of readiness, or stages of change construct, to be useful in determining which patients would reach and sustain viral suppression (Enriquez, Gore, O'Connor, & McKinsey, 2004). Last, a prediction model using the TTM constructs correctly identified 82 percent of patients who would discontinue interferon β-1a (Avenox) use for multiple sclerosis and identified with 81 percent accuracy those who would stay on the treatment regimen (Berger, Hudmon, & Liang, 2004).

This growing body of evidence supports the use of the TTM across multiple disease states in medication compliance.

OTHER MODELS

While the previously discussed five theoretical cognitive models have garnered the greatest amount of attention in the medication compliance literature, they are by no means the only models one should consider. The literature is replete with numerous conceptual models, single construct investigations, and atheoretical interventions evaluated to improve the medication compliance of our patients. While a comprehensive review of all the approaches in the literature is beyond the scope of this chapter, there are a few other notable models of which one should be aware.

Rotter's Social Learning Theory (1954) was an adaptation of the original model that was developed to explain how animals and humans learn by imitating the behavior of others. Rotter believed that our behavior is influenced by observing the actions of others and that positive and negative reinforcement of behaviors will occur based on the outcomes of observed events. The main tenet of the social learning theory is that behavior is based on an individual's expectancy that the action will lead to a particular reinforcement and the extent that the reinforcement is valued. The construct locus of control was developed in this model as a form of generalized expectancy and makes the distinction between internal control over a situation versus external control over events. This construct has been widely adopted and applied in health psychology. Other constructs of the model include health value and social support.

The protection motivation theory was developed to understand the reactions to fear. It describes adaptive and maladaptive coping to a health threat through the processes of threat appraisal and coping appraisal (Rogers, 1975). Threat appraisal is governed by the individual's perceived susceptibility and severity to the illness while coping appraisal is the product of the individual's belief that a behavior will decrease the health threat (action-outcome efficacy) and the individual's belief in accomplishing the behavior (self-efficacy). These two processes form the intention to perform an adaptive response (protection motivation) or a maladaptive response. The protection motivation model is often applied to an intention to perform a health protective behavior or to avoid a health compromising behavior.

Last, the self-regulation theory is a series of models that are founded on the metatheory that cognitive factors are significant contributors to health behaviors. The concept of self-regulation has been defined in a number of ways, but a common definition is "a systematic process of human behavior toward the achievement of established goals . . . Overall definitions tend to embody the basic ingredients of goal setting, steering process and strategies, feedback, and self-evaluation" (Zeidner, Boekaerts, & Pintrich, 2000, p. 750). While the self-regulation models presented in the literature differ in their details, they all are grounded in three principles: self-monitoring of health behavior, adoption of goals to direct the individual's efforts and strategies for achieving the goals, and self-evaluation that incorporates motivational incentives and social support to sustain the healthy behavior (Bandura, 2005). The overall aim is to close the difference between where one is currently and where one would ideally like to be.

CONCLUSIONS

This chapter has provided an overview of some of the most important behavioral models that have been used in medication compliance research and presented in the literature. The use of the determinants from these behavioral models can serve as an underpinning for sound medication compliance interventions and should allow researchers in this area to create programs that can be adapted and applied across a number of disease states. It is believed that these models offer an important way to achieve the goals of producing better outcomes to treatment and improving the health and quality of life for our patients.

Whether further development of these models will lead to improved results and increased understanding remains to be seen. As our knowledge of effective interventions for our patients continues to grow, we can apply this knowledge to the direct benefit of our patients.

REFERENCES

Abraham, C., Clift, S., & Grabowski, P. (1999). Cognitive predictors of adherence to malaria prophylaxis regimens on return from a malarious region: A prospective study. *Soc Sci Med, 48*(11): 1641-1654.

Adams, J., & Scott, J. (2000). Predicting medication adherence in severe mental disorders. *Acta Psychiatr Scand, 101*(2): 119-124.

Ajzen, I. (1985). From intentions to actions: A theory of planned behavior. In Kuhl, J. & Beckmann, J. (Eds.), *Action control: From cognition to behavior* (pp. 11-38). New York, NY: Springer Publishing Company.

Ajzen, I., & Fishbein, M. (1980). *Understanding attitudes and predicting social behavior* (p. 119). Englewood Cliffs, NJ: Prentice Hall.

Alogna, M. (1980). Perception of severity of disease and health locus of control in compliant and noncompliant diabetic patients. *Diabetes Care, 3*(4): 533-534.

Bandura, A. (1977). Self-efficacy: Toward a unifying theory of behavioral change. *Psychological Review, 84*(2): 191-215.

Bandura, A. (1982). Self-efficacy mechanism in human agency. *American Psychologist, 37*(2): 122-147.

Bandura, A. (1986). *Social foundations of thought and action: A social cognitive theory* (p. 277). Englewood Cliffs, NJ: Prentice Hall, Inc.

Bandura, A. (2004). Health promotion by social cognitive means. *Health Education and Behavior, 31:* 143-164.

Bandura, A. (2005). The primacy of self-regulation in health promotion. *Applied Psychology: An International Review, 54*(2): 245-254.

Becker, M. H. (1974). The health belief model and sick role behavior. *Health Educ Monogr, 2:* 409-419.

Becker, M. H. (1976). The role of the patient: Social and psychological factors in noncompliance. In Lasagna, L. (Ed.), *Patient compliance* (p. 135). Mt. Kisco, NY: Futura publishing.

Becker, M. H., Maiman, L. A., Kirscht, J. P., Haefner, D. P., & Drachman, R. H. (1977). The Health Belief Model and prediction of dietary compliance: A field experiment. *J Health Soc Behav, 18*(4): 348-366.

Berger, B. A., Hudmon, K. S., & Liang, H. (2004). Predicting treatment discontinuation among patients with multiple sclerosis: Application of the transtheoretical model of change. *JAPhA, 44*(4): 445-454.

Brownlee-Duffeck, M., Peterson, L., Eidsen, M., & Delamater, A. (1987). The role of health beliefs in the regimen adherence and metabolic control of adolescents and adults with diabetes mellitus. *J Consult Clin Psych, 55*(2): 139-144.

Brubaker, R. G., Prue, D. M., & Rychtarik, A. (1987). Determinants of disulfiram acceptance among alcohol patients: A test of the theory of reasoned action. *Addictive Behaviors, 12*(1): 43-51.

Budd, R. J., Hughes, I. C., & Smith, J. A. (1996). Health beliefs and compliance with antipsychotic medication. *Br J Clin Psychol, 35*(Pt 3): 393-397.

Cerkoney, K. A., & Hart, L. K. (1980). The relationship between the health belief model and compliance of persons with diabetes mellitus. *Diabetes Care, 3*(5): 594-598.

Chao, J. (2004). The relationship between depressive symptoms and oral antihyperglycemic medication adherence. Dissertation Abstracts International: Section B: The Sciences & Engineering, *Univ Microfilms International, 65:* 2891.

Clark, N. M., & Becker, M. H. (1998). Theoretical models and strategies for improving adherence and disease management. In Shumaker, S. A. & Schron, E. B. (Eds.), *Handbook of health behavior change* (2nd ed.) (pp. 5-32). Springer.

Cochran, S. D., & Gitlin, M. J. (1988). Attitudinal correlates of lithium compliance in bipolar affective disorders. *Journal of Nervous & Mental Disease, 176*(8): 457-464.

Connelly, C. E., Davenport, Y. B., & Nurnberger, J. (1982). Adherence to treatment regimen in a lithium carbonate clinic. *Arch Gen Psychiatry, 39*(5): 585-588.

Conner, M., Black, K. et al. (1998). Understanding drug compliance in a psychiatric population: An application of the Theory of Planned Behaviour. *Psych Health Med, 3*(3): 337-344.

Conner, M., & Norman, P. (1996a). *Predicting health behaviour: Research and practice with social cognition models* (pp. 23-30). Buckingham, UK: Open University Press.

Conner, M., & Norman, P. (1996b). *The role of social cognition in health behaviours. Predicting health behaviour: Research and practice with social cognition models* (pp. 1-22). UK Open University Press.

Cook, C. L., & Perri, M. (2004). Single-item vs multiple-item measures of stage of change in compliance with prescribed medications. *Psychol Rep, 94*(1): 115-124.

Cook, C. L., & University of Georgia (2002). *Validation of the transtheoretical model in medication compliance behavior* (p. xii, 132 leaves). Doctoral Dissertation, The University of Georgia, Athens, Georgia.

Costa, L. L. (1999). Association of hospitalized heart failure patients' intention to manage the therapeutic regimen with postdischarge health behaviors and outcomes. (therapy outcomes). *Dissertation Abstracts International: Section B: The Sciences & Engineering, Univ Microfilms International, 60:* 1527.

DiClemente, C. C., Prochaska, J. O., Fairhurst, S. K., Velicer, W. F., Velasquez, M. M., & Rossi, J. S. (1991). The process of smoking cessation: An analysis of precontemplation, contemplation, and preparation stages of change. *J Consult Clin Psychol, 59*(2): 295-304.

DiIorio, C., Hennessy, M., & Manteuffel, L. (1996). Epilepsy self-management: A test of a theoretical model. *Nurs Res, 45*(4): 211-217.

Enriquez, M., Gore, P. A. J., O'Connor, M. C., & McKinsey, D. S. (2004). Assessment of readiness for adherence by HIV-positive males who had previously failed treatment. *JANAC, 15*(1): 42-49.

Fincham, J. E., & Wertheimer, A. I. (1985). Using the health belief model to predict initial drug therapy defaulting. *Soc Sci Med, 20*(1): 101-105.

Fiske, S. T., & Taylor, S. E. (1991). *Social cognition* (2nd ed.) (p. 450). New York: McGraw-Hill Book Company.

Grimley, D. M., Prochaska, G. E., Velicer, W. F., Galavotti, C., Cabral, R. J., & Lansky, A. (1996). Cross-validation of measures assessing decisional balance and self-efficacy for condom use. *Am J of Health Behav, 20*(6): 406-416.

Hochbaum, G. (1958). Public participation in medical screening programs: A sociopsychological study. *Public Health Service Publication.* Washington, DC: United States Government Printing Office.

Johnson, S. S., Grimley, D. M., & Prochaska, J. O. (1998). Prediction of adherence using the transtheoretical model: Implications for pharmacy care practice. *Journal of Social and Administrative Pharmacy, 15*(3): 135-148.

Kalichman, S. C., Cain, D., Fuhrel, A., Eaton, L., Di Fonzo, K., & Ertl, T. (2005). Assessing medication adherence self-efficacy among low-literacy patients: Development of a pictographic visual analogue scale. *Health Educ Res, 20*(1): 24-35.

Kavanagh, D. J., Gooley, S., & Wilson, P. (1993). Prediction of adherence and control in diabetes. *J Behav Med, 16*(5): 509-522.

Kelly, G. R., Mamon, J. A., & Scott, J. (1987). Utility of the health belief model in examining medication compliance among psychiatric outpatients. *Soc Sci Med, 25*(11): 1205-1211.

Kirscht, J. P. (1974). The health belief model and illness behavior. *Health Educ Monogr, 2:* 387-408.

Lorish, C. D., Richards, B., & Brown, S. (1990). Perspective of the patient with rheumatoid arthritis on issues related to missed medication. *Arthritis Care Res, 3*(2): 78-84.

Maiman, L. A., & Becker, M. H. (1974). The health belief model: Origins and correlates in psychological theory. *Health Educ Monogr, 2:* 336-353.

McCaul, K. D., Glasgow, R. E., & Schafer, L. (1987). Diabetes regimen behaviors: Predicting adherence. *Medical Care, 25*(9): 868-881.

Miller, P., Wikoff, R., & Hiatt, A. (1992). Fishbein's model of reasoned action and compliance behavior of hypertensive patients. *Nurs Res, 41*(2): 104-109.

Pan, P. C., & Tantam, D. (1989). Clinical characteristics, health beliefs and compliance with maintenance treatment: A comparison between regular and irregular attenders at a depot clinic. *Acta Psychiatr Scand, 79*(6): 564-570.

Peak, H. (1955). Attitude and motivation. In Jones, M. R. (Ed.), *Nebraska symposium on motivation* (pp. 149-189). Lincoln, NE: University of Nebraska.

Prochaska, J. O., DiClemente, C. C., Velicer, W., Ginpil, S., & Norcross, T. (1985). Predicting change in smoking status for self-changers. *Addict Behav, 10*(4): 395-406.

Prochaska, J. O., Velicer, W. F., Guadagnoli, E., & Rossi, J. (1991). Patterns of change: Dynamic typology applied to smoking cessation. *Multivariate Behavioral Research, 26*(1): 83-107.

Prochaska, J. O., Velicer, W. F., Rossi, J. S., Goldstein, M. G., Marcus, B. H., & Rakowski, W. (1994). Stages of change and decisional balance for 12 problem behaviors. *Health Psychol, 13*(1): 39-46.

Putman, H. P. (2002). Knowledge, health beliefs, attitude, and behavioral intention as predictors of compliance with prescribed treatment regimens in rural Appalachian adults diagnosed with asthma. *Dissertation Abstracts International: Section B: The Sciences & Engineering, Univ Microfilms International, 63:* 742.

Resnick, B., Wehren, L., & Orwig, D. (2003). Reliability and validity of the self-efficacy and outcome expectations for osteoporosis medication adherence scales. *Orthop Nurs, 22*(2): 139-147.

Ried, L. D., & Christensen, D. B. (1988). Psychosocial perspective in the explanation of patients drug taking behavior. *Social Science and Medicine, 27*(3): 277-285.

Ried, L. D., Oleen, M. A., Martinson, O. B., & Pluhar, R. (1985). Explaining intention to comply with antihypertensive regimens: Utility of health beliefs and the theory of reasoned action. *J Soc Admin Pharm, 3*(2): 42-52.

Rogers, R. W. (1975). A protection motivation theory of fear appeals and attitude change. *J Psychy: Interdisc App, 91*(1): 93-114.

Rosenstock, I. M. (1966). Why people use health services. *Mil Mem Fund Q, 44:* 94-124.

Rossi, S. R., & Rossi, J. S. (1999). Concepts and theoretical models applicable to risk reduction. In Jairath, N. (Ed.), *Coronary heart disease and risk factor management: A Nursing perspective* (pp. 47-69). Orlando, FL: W.B. Saunders.

Scott, J. (2002). Using Health Belief Models to understand the efficacy-effectiveness gap for mood stabilizer treatments. *Neuropsychobiology, 46* (Suppl 1): 13-15.

Senecal, C., Nouwen, A., & White, D. (2000). Motivation and dietary self-care in adults with diabetes: Are self-efficacy and autonomous self-regulation complementary or competing constructs? *Health Psychol, 19*(5): 452-457.

Smith, S. R., Rublein, J. C., Marcus, C., Brock, T. P., & Chesney, M. A. (2003). A medication self-management program to improve adherence to HIV therapy regimens. *Pat Educ Couns, 50*(2): 187-199.

Stroebe, W., & Stroebe, M. S. (1995). *Social psychology and health* (pp. 120-137). St. Paul, MN: Brooks/Cole Publishing.

Taal, E., Rasker, J. J., Seydel, F., & Wiegman, O. (1993). Health status, adherence with health recommendations, self-efficacy and social support in patients with rheumatoid arthritis. *Pat Educ Couns, 20*(2): 63-76.

Terry, D. J., Gallois, C., & McCamish, M. (1993). *The theory of reasoned action: Its application to AIDS-preventive behaviour* (pp. 217-234). London, UK: Routledge.

Tuldra, A., Fumaz, C. R., Ferrer, M. J., Bayes, R., Arno, A., Balague, M., et al. (2000). Prospective randomized two-arm controlled study to determine the efficacy of a specific intervention to improve long-term adherence to highly active antiretroviral therapy. *J Acquir Immune Defic Syndr, 25*(3): 221-228.

Tutty, S., Simon, G., & Ludman, F. (2000). Telephone counseling as an adjunct to antidepressant treatment in the primary care system. A pilot study. *Eff Clin Pract, 3*(4): 170-178.

Velicer, W. F., DiClemente, C. C., Prochaska, J.O., & Brandenburg, N. (1985). Decisional balance measure for assessing and predicting smoking status. *J Pers Soc Psychol, 48*(5): 1279-1289.

Velicer, W. F., DiClemente, C. C., Rossi, J. S., & Prochaska, J. O. (1990). Relapse situations and self-efficacy: An integrative model. *Addictive Behaviors, 15*(3): 271-283.

Willey, C., Redding, C., Stafford, J., Garfield, F., Geletko, S., Flanigan, T., et al. (2000). Stages of change for adherence with medication regimens for chronic disease: Development and validation of a measure. *Clin Ther, 22*(7): 858-871.

Zeidner, M., Boekaerts, M., & Pintrich, P. R. (2000). Self-regulation: Directions and challenges for future research. In Boekaerts, M. & Pintrich, P. R. (Eds.), *Handbook of self-regulation* (pp. 749-768). San Diego, CA: Academic Press.

Chapter 7

Methods to Impact Patient Compliance

It is one thing to talk about medications, their positive effects, potential adverse effects, but it is difficult to follow through and be compliant with the drugs that should be taken. Compliance with medications is extremely difficult for many patients and for caregivers taking care of patients and loved ones. Fitting in specific dosing times during otherwise hectic days can be a challenge for anyone.

TYPES OF IMPACTS ON COMPLIANCE

There are three basic types of impacts on compliance. They are organizational, educational, and behavioral (Dunbar, Marshall, & Hovell, 1979). Within these broad guidelines, there are many types of interventions.

Organizational Aspects of Care

Organizational impacts include the way care is provided for patients. How are the clinics where patients seek care structured? If patients are able to park, readily move from an automobile to the pharmacy, and through the pharmacy to the prescription counter, they are more likely to have convenient access to the pharmacist for questions or assistance. After receiving physician care, is it easy for patients to obtain prescription medications? Do pharmacies provide convenience and ease of access for patients? Is it a hassle to obtain prescriptions? Do patients have to work through a maze of aisles and barriers

Patient Compliance with Medications: Issues and Opportunities
© 2007 by The Haworth Press, Inc. All rights reserved.
doi:10.1300/5365_07

to reach the pharmacy? Is it convenient for patients to follow through on the care that has been recommended for them? If not, patients may be less inclined to even bother to have prescriptions filled or refilled.

Patients may be given incentives to use mail-order pharmacies, and may find the process more convenient (Thomas, 2003). Chronic medications may be logical candidate drugs to obtain from mail-order pharmacies. Problems may occur with the need for acute medications and patients being unaware of the differences between acute and chronic conditions. Medications such as antibiotics, medications for allergy symptoms, or pain-relief medications are needed by patients quickly, and waiting for arrival from the mail-order pharmacy may be counterproductive. But if patients are unsure which medications are for chronic conditions, and which are for acute conditions, mail-order pharmacies may not be the best option for them.

The need to have ease of access to a pharmacist for questions is just as important as the physical manner in which patients receive their medications, There is nothing worse than trying to ask a pharmacist a question, and not be able to talk with the pharmacist without an extensive series of explanations or buttons on a phone to wade through. Errant pharmacists making medication errors have been a source of diminishing patient compliance as well (Hughes & Ortiz, 2005). *Also, the integrity and ethical issues surrounding pharmacists have reached a wider audience than the pharmacy profession would like* (see Figure 7.1).

Pharmacists, because of their accessibility, are in an ideal position to influence long-term adherence on the part of patients (Hoek, 2003). The importance of pharmacists has been shown to improve compliance of numerous patients with varying diseases: hypertensives (Blenkinsopp, Phelan, Bourne, & Dakhil, 2000), asthmatics (Cordina, McElnay, & Hughes, 2001; Schulz et al., 2001), and transplant patients (Chisholm, Mulloy, Jagadeesan, & DiPiro, 2001).

Educational Aspects of Care

The educational aspects of care relate to the advice and counseling received from pharmacists. The more one knows about the health care received in general, and specifically, the more aware one is about the

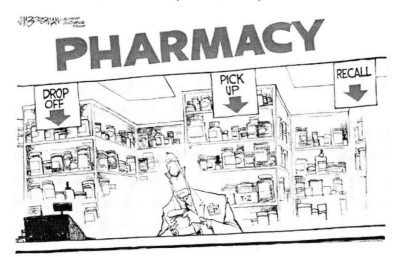

FIGURE 7.1. "Integrity on Back Order." (*Source:* Integrity on Back Order, Jim Brogman, *Cincinnati Enquirer,* © Reprinted with special permission of King Features Syndicate.)

medications that are taken, the more likely would be one's compliance (Haynes, McDonald, & Garg, 2002; Sabaté, 2003).

Patients can receive advice and counseling from physicians, nurses, or pharmacists. Verbal advice is helpful in allowing patients to understand the need to be compliant. It is important that the verbal counseling that patients receive be concise, informative, and specific to patient needs (McDonald, Garg, & Haynes, 2002). If the information provided is personalized and individualized, patients may be more inclined to realize the benefits from drug therapy (Peterson, Takiya, & Finley, 2003).

Information may also be provided through a leaflet that is received with prescriptions. This written information is general in nature and is not specific to a patient. They provide blanket information about a drug or a class of drugs and are printed off as a drug within the specific class dispensed to anyone else receiving the drug. These written leaflets usually contain segments such as the following:

• The name of the medication
• What the uses of the drug commonly are

- How you should take the medication
- Some common side effects

The lack of adequate information for patients receive concerning the drugs they take has prompted the federal government to become involved in mandating the provision of information to patients. The OBRA '90 guidelines stipulate that certain information be offered to patients among other tenets. Some pharmacies go above and beyond the minimum requirements specified in these guidelines. Others simply follow the basic letter of the law.

These governmental efforts are not lacking in cause; patients simply do not understand enough about the drugs they take. Efforts to institute mandated patient package inserts (PPIs) in the 1970s and 1980s were aimed at the lack of patient drug knowledge and receipt of such from health professionals.

However, written information alone is not the answer. There needs to be individualized assessment and interventions aimed at particular and specific patient needs. The usual side-effect information that is provided in these leaflets, although it may be useful, is often very limited. The worth of these leaflets has been subject to much discussion and analysis. The information is inadequate if the leaflet is all the counseling received about prescriptions. If it complements what has been told verbally by a pharmacist or physician, the written information can be useful supplemental material.

The most useful type of information that patients receive the most benefit from is a combination of verbal and written information (Fincham, 1998). Here face-to-face counseling can be augmented with written materials to reinforce the information transmitted verbally. The important party in this counseling scenario is always the patient. Patients must be ready to hear and read what is meant for them; if they are too busy to wait at the pharmacy to be counseled, a time should be set up with the pharmacist that is more convenient for them. This can be either in person or via the telephone. If medications are dispensed by a mail-order pharmacy, the pharmacy must provide a 1-800 toll free phone number for patients to call in order to have questions answered. This is a right, and patients should expect no less than all the information necessary, whether in person or via the phone.

Behavioral Aspects of Care

The most difficult task any of us has is the need to change our behaviors. There are over 250 factors related to compliant behavior (Fincham & Wertheimer, 1985). Of this number, some are certainly no doubt behavioral in nature. Patient compliance is an individual-specific response by patients that is variable and often unpredictable in any number of differing patients and/or diseases. Attitude makes a tremendous impact on the outcomes of drug therapies. If a patient feels that drugs will not work, or that the physician or pharmacist is not capable of providing care, the chances are good that they will be less than optimally compliant. By the same token, if one believes in their caregivers and their recommendations, they have a better chance of success in complying with medical therapies.

If patients are satisfied with the care that they receive, they are more likely to have positive outcomes and have more of a chance to be compliant with prescribed medications. Physician communication style and patient satisfaction with care are both positively correlated with higher rates of patient compliance (Bultman & Svarstad, 2000). The more the care provided in a patient-centered approach, the more likely the patient satisfaction and compliance with recommendations (Stevenson, Barry, Britten, Barber, & Bradley, 2000).

The more knowledge one has of the disease and the drugs that may be used to treat the ailment, the better are the chances of being compliant. It is important for patients to learn as much as possible about their disease(s), read all that they can about the disease, and always ask questions to obtain more information. Just because it is difficult to change it does not mean that it cannot happen.

SPECIFIC WAYS TO IMPROVE COMPLIANCE

The most crucial consideration to keep in mind with regard to patient compliance is that impacts upon noncompliant patients must be individualized. What works for one patient may or may not be useful for someone else. Individuals are just that; so impacts upon noncompliance must also be individualized.

Calendars

These calendars can be as simple or as complex as one wishes. The idea is to mark when medications are to be taken on a regular calendar, date book, or printed monthly calendar with the days of the week listed on the sheet. There are two ways one can do this:

- Write on the calendar when medications *are* to be taken, or
- Write on the calendar when the medication *has been* taken.

This calendar type of reminder alerts patients to when they are to take the medication and lets them indicate that they have taken the medication. If patients are to take some medications on an as-needed basis, have them write down the times and quantity taken each day.

The use of calendar packaging has been used by some manufacturers for many years. Oral contraceptive tablets have traditionally been packaged with a calendar-blister pack design for decades. This allows the woman to see on a daily basis whether she has taken the tablet she is to take. Also, some steroid medications have been packaged with a calendar blister setup. This allows the patient to see how many tablets they are to take on a daily basis, and how many they in fact have taken that day. An example of this packaging concept is the Decadron Dosepak, which contains dexamethasone tablets that should be taken on a tapered-dose basis. This is a dosage regimen that might be prescribed for a patient stung by a bee or wasp, or by one who has suffered an allergic reaction to a substance. Tapered in the sense that tablets are taken on a decreasing-quantity and daily-dosage level for a period of time until the regimen is completed. This allows the patient to take the right number of tablets for the right period of time, thus avoiding either an underdose or overdose of the medication.

Diaries

Using a diary approach is very similar to the calendar option, except that one chronicles the drugs that are taken on a daily basis and lists how they feel that day and possibly the reactions that they are having with the medications. These reactions can be either positive or negative. For example, the patient can list the dose of insulin or the oral hypoglycemic drug either administered or consumed, and then list what the blood sugar levels might be, or how they have felt during the day. Maintaining such a journal allows the patient to reflect back on changes in health that might have first appeared in something that they have written. They also might track blood pressure daily and write the dosage of the medications taken that day.

If they are taking a drug to treat depression, they can write down the times that they have taken a drug to treat it, and list their feelings for the day. How have they been able to sleep? Are they anxious for no reason? Do they feel downhearted sad and blue to a great extent? Have them chronicle their feelings and commit them to writing. Then, the next time that they see their physician, they can report on how they have been doing since they were last seen. This gives a reference point to discern whether they are gaining or losing ground, and how they have been feeling. It can be overwhelming to try to summarize from memory day-to-day feelings without some frame of reference for a guide. Finally, if they have forgotten to take a medication, they can easily write this fact down as well in a diary. The diary does not have to be a sophisticated or expensive volume; it can simply be a collection of sheets of paper that they have organized in a systematic fashion somewhere.

Packaging

The ease of opening a container may seem an inconsequential act. But if you cannot open a container in order to remove and administer a dose, it becomes a major impediment to compliance. This is an important issue for many seniors, as well as others who cannot open a vial without some amount of difficulty. There are situations where people find one container that they can open and place all of their medications in this one container. This is not the best way to deal with the problem. Patients should ask their pharmacist about options for obtaining their medications in a container that they can open. It may be that the prescription vials are too small for them to get a good grip and thus they cannot maneuver the container to open it. Pharmacists can provide a larger container or one that is longer and that can be grasped and held while the cap is being opened on the top of the vial.

Nonchild-resistant Closures

Patients can also request that all of their prescriptions be dispensed with a nonchild-resistant closure. This request can be on an item-by-item basis, or on a "blanket" basis, by signing a form that requests that all containers be dispensed as nonchild-resistant containers. Some vials have reversible caps that can serve either as child-resistant or nonchild-resistant closures. This is a solution that a pharmacist can easily provide. Some mail-order pharmacies also send extra caps that are not child resistant with each prescription that they mail out for ease of patient use.

If patients have young children or grandchildren in the house, they may want containers to be child resistant. This is their choice, and pharmacies dispense medications in a child-resistant fashion; they are legally obligated to do so, unless asked otherwise by the patient.

One can really be in a sticky situation, figuratively and literally, if they have a prescription for a liquid medication in syrup form. The sugar content can coalesce at the ridge of the top of the bottle and form a sticky barrier that makes opening the container difficult to say the least. Patients can be told to wipe the top with a clean cloth or towel after each opening, so the syrup never has the chance to build up at the top and prevent ease of access. It will work best if the cloth is wetted first to help clear off the liquid. A paper towel or napkin is probably not the best method, since the paper will stick to the syrupy liquid and attached as well. Here again, a pharmacist can provide patients with containers that are not child resistant for prescriptions that are liquids or solutions.

The use of specialized devices to administer and remind patients about dosing is not new. Please see Figure 7.2, displaying a dosing spoon with time indicator for administration of the next dose on the handle. This compliance timing spoon (U.S. Patent 1,619,878; Issued March 8, 1927) was patented by H. D. Morgan and F. P. Bushey in 1927 and marketed as the "Next-Dose" Spoon. There are lines on the spoon indicating half and one teaspoon measure points. There is scant mention of compliance in the literature 100 years ago, but pharmacies and patients found these devices to be useful. For the pharmacist, advertising on the spoon provided a reminder of their services, and for the patient, a reminder was present on the body of the spoon to

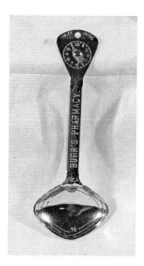

FIGURE 7.2. "Compliance Dosing Spoon." (*Source:* Photo: Ms. Wendy E. Giminski, computer graphics artist, The University of Georgia. Copyright Jack E. Fincham, PhD. Compliance Spoon Collection, The University of Georgia. All rights reserved.)

remind them of the next dosing time. Most medications were in liquid form, and a device to help accurately measure liquid, elixir, tonic, suspensions was a highly sought-after item. Prior to this time, in the late nineteenth century, a similar dosing spoon was patented in Great Britain. The difference in the spoons rested with the metal resin used in the two devices; the U.K. device was a higher-grade silver product, while the U.S. spoon was an amalgamated mixture that allowed mass production with an accompanying economy of scale.

Inhalers, nebulizers, and specialized sprays are available in only one type of container. Thus a pharmacist cannot provide alternative containers for these medications. If one has trouble accessing these medications, a pharmacist can be asked to help in making their access as easy as possible.

Divided Containers: Specialized Pill Boxes

There are several companies that market divided "pill" containers. These containers have seven, fourteen, or twenty-eight separated segments where patients can place a day's, two week's, or a month's worth of medications inside. These divided pill boxes allow the patient to see what has been taken on a daily basis and allows the patient to place the required doses in a container in an organized fashion.

There are also various sizes for the daily segments so that a person who takes numerous drugs daily can place them all in the container. These containers are specifically designed to keep medications dry and have closures that help to ensure the medications stay fresh. I have to stress that these types of containers are a much better option than trying to place medications in any type of separated containers. This author has seen medications placed in fly fishing lure separated boxes. These are *not* containers recommended for use as medication separators!

Medicine-on-Time[1] is an innovative company that provides a system of packaging and labeling that quickly identifies the dosing time for medications, and provides a heat- and water-resistant compartment that allows all the drugs for a certain dosing interval to be packaged together for ease of patient consumption. There is also a high-capacity container for holding up to twelve dosing units. This technology has been very useful for both patients and for caregivers. Caregivers are able to distribute complex dosing regimens in a color-coded and secure fashion through the Medicine-on-Time system.

One retail line of medication containers is the Ezy-dose container products. Forgettingthepill.com also sells a complete line of these types of containers. Some containers even have timers to alert you to when you need to take your medications. There are some tablets that should not be placed in these types of containers—one such drug is nitroglycerin. Nitroglycerin tablets are taken to alleviate cardiac pain (angina pectoris). These tablets are very sensitive to light and heat and moisture. Nitroglycerin is just too susceptible to environmental changes and should always be left in the manufacturer-supplied containers. The stability of these tablets is just too important to risk transfer to another container.

Another innovative device to aid patient compliance is the MedivoxRx talking prescription vial (Rex—The Talking Pill Bottle). This is a prescription vial that contains a device to record prescription-label information (drug name, date, directions, etc.). In a study of twenty-five visually impaired patients at a Veterans Administration

(VA) facility, a total of twenty patients understood the directions, but only fifteen strongly agreed that the voice was easily understood (Englehardt, Allnatt, Mariano, & Gao, 2001). This problem with understanding the voice could easily be remedied by a more distinctive recorded message(s) (Englehardt et al., 2001).

Electronic Monitors

Some patients are helped by memory-reminding devices. There are several devices on the market that can help remind a person to take medications on schedule. These items stimulate patients to take medications as directed. The complexity of these devices varies from simple to complex. For example, forgettingthepill.com sells a device with up to thirty-one possible alarms per day for dosing reminders. This might be a stretch expecting patients to set so many alarms to help with their medication-taking needs when they have trouble taking prescribed doses as it is.

GETTING INTO THE HABIT OF COMPLYING

A good habit to acquire is compliance nearing 100 percent. There are certain things that one can do to help remember to take medications. One suggestion would be timing and grouping as options for consideration.

Timing

Patients brush their teeth several times a day, and the timing of this activity is similar from day to day. They can take medications at an approximate time as this helps them to remember to comply and to get into the habit of doing so. Taking their "statin" drug, a high blood pressure medication, and/or a drug to treat heart failure at the same time as they brush their teeth may help them place the taking of these drugs in a rhythm. It will be so routine for them that it would become second nature to take medications at that time. Are there other routine activities in daily life that can be paired with medication taking? If patients need to take medications with them to their worksite, they can place the medication containers in a spot that they can use as an anchor to help remind them of the next dosing interval. This might be a lunch-box, desk drawer that is accessed routinely, or in a purse or briefcase. By coupling normal daily activities with medication taking, patients can begin to help themselves become better compliers.

Grouping

It is daunting to consider drug regimens that require complex dos-ing, for example, to take one tablet daily, another twice a day, a third three times daily, a fourth four times daily, and perhaps yet another every four hours. If they then have a medication that is to be taken on an as-needed basis, it is possible to see how quickly someone can be-come confused about what they should take and when they should take it. Without trying to oversimplify a very complex situation, there are some things that one can do to help organize this. If it is possible, the doses for the morning regimens can be taken at the same time. They may have to take numerous medications at the same time. But, it is felt that this is a better situation than trying to remember to take nu-merous medications at different times in the morning. The same grouping activity can be done at around lunchtime, supper time, and at bedtime. If they are to take a medication every six hours, can they combine this medication with others that they take three or four times a day? Patients can be assisted to develop a method of ensuring that they remember to take the doses that they are supposed to take.

Finally, if they take medications on an as-needed basis, they can take these at a similar time as they take the other medications that are routinely taken. So, if they take a medication for pain on an as-needed basis, take it with others so that they can remember that they have taken it, and can track the number that they take daily.

Count Backward to Move Forward

If patients are at a point where they simply cannot remember whether they have taken all the drugs that they are supposed to take, help them help themselves with some facts. Usually medications are dispensed on a thirty-day basis. They might want to count the number of tablets or capsules that they have left in the container and count the number of days since they have had the prescription filled. They might be able to figure out how many units they should have taken and figure out how many are reamaining. Then they can move ahead to decide whether they should take the dose or not. They can empty the container of tablets or capsules into a bowl, count them and place them back in the container, and determine whether they need to take another medication or not.

Buddy System

It is also useful to have someone else help them remember to take their medications. This may be a friend, a colleague, or a family member. This technique is doubly helpful if they are taking a drug that might affect their mental state, and affect their memory in a negative fashion. If their medications affect their memory, have them understand that they do not need to feel that this is some flaw in their character. Many medications have the potential to do this. Recognizing that it might happen, they can have their friends or loved ones help them remember, and always make the best of the situation.

OTHER CONSIDERATIONS

Many other devices have been used to try and improve patient compliance. These range from prescriber order entry by physicians (Segarra, DeStefano, & Davis, 1991) with the goal of decreasing prescription-processing time and increasing the opportunities for pharmacists to work with patients. Computer-generated reminder charts for patients (Forcino, 1991) and various caps and counter-devices have also been tried.

E-Prescribing

Automatic prescription order entry, also termed e-prescribing (electronic prescribing) occurs when the physician enters a prescription information automatically, and it is then transmitted to the pharmacy for dispensing. There is nothing that the patient needs to do other than simply go to the pharmacy to pick up his or her medications. This has the potential to decrease errors in prescribing and dispensing, and makes it easier for the patient to comply. The Medicare Modernization Act of 2003 has e-prescribing as a component to be standardized by 2009.

Tablet Splitting

This has been both acclaimed and criticized as a method to increase compliance. It is acclaimed because theoretically by making a medication go twice as far, patients will be more inclined to be compliant because it is less expensive for them to comply with their medication regimens. However, the use of a tablet splitter to enable economic savings by dividing a higher-dose tablet into two smaller doses was found to discourage patients from complying because of confusion (Carr-Lopez, Allett, & Morse, 1995). There are also many drugs in dosage forms that should not be split. These dosage forms include capsule formulations, extended release or controlled release medications. The drugs in these extended release formulations are meant to be dispersed over an eight- to twelve-hour period. Also, there are some drugs that are enteric-coated formulations that should not be sliced open. Drugs that are enteric-coated are meant to dissolve in the less acidic (basic) environment of the intestines rather than the stomach. These drugs are formulated as enteric-coated so that you will not experience a stomach upset when taking the medication. Drugs that cause stomach upset formulated in the enteric-coated form will not cause the stomach upset when dissolved in the intestine. Aspirin, some laxatives (bisacodyl—Dulcolax), and other products are enteric-coated to minimize stomach upset. As an aside, if bisacodyl were not enteric-coated, and swallowed as is, stomach upset would be a certain outcome of the dosing. It also comes in a suppository formulation for quicker action for some who prefer this route of administration.

Specialized Caps

The use of a notched, clicking cap for prescription medications has been shown to increase compliance (Perri, Martin, & Pritchard, 1995). These caps are a visual reminder for when to take your medication, and a way of telling that you have taken your medication. Caps imbedded with electronic devices that can then download information to a computer to track compliance have been used as compliance-detecting and recording tools (Urquhart, 1993). The cost of some of these items might be prohibitive for many patients and contain too much technology to be useful for many people. Other electronic devices can measure removal compliance from blister-packaged doses (Wingender & Kuppers, 1993).

Blister Packaging

Blister packaging is a process whereby the medications that are taken are heat-sealed in a small compartment, placed in an accessible card, and are easy to extract at the time of dosing. Here again, one has a visual reminder of what is to be taken, and what has or has not been taken. Blister packaging and compliance packaging have been used to enhance compliance (Tiano, 1994). Blister packaging and unit-of-use materials are extensively used for prescription medications elsewhere in the world (Forcinio, 1993). Some blister packs are sometimes referred to as "bingo" cards due to the similar shape and visual appearance of the medication cards.

Tablets are rarely moved from one large container to a smaller container elsewhere in the world. It is a uniquely American phenomenon. This is *not* the best way to get medications to the consumer. Due to the visual reminder aspects of unit-of-use packaging, patients have the potential to be more compliant. However, unit-of-use packaging is not without controversy, it has in fact been criticized for lack of standardization between products and manufacturers that can confuse patients (Rigby, 2002).

SUMMARY

In summary the important thing to note is that whatever works best for a patient is what they should use. They may also combine several or more of the aforementioned suggestions to help to greater extent. Basically, if the calendar combined with the divided pill box approach works best for them, then so be it. Patients are the final determiners of what might be best for them. They might also try several aforementioned suggestions to see whether any of these works better for them for their particular needs.

For the most part, with regard to compliance-enhancing strategies—the more things that can be done the better the chances success. Patients can be encouraged to combine a memory enhancer or behavioral cue with a container aid or a calendar or diary to further help their possibilities of successful compliance. Enhancing compliance is more art than science, and more trial and error than smooth precision. Success may be frustratingly difficult to achieve, but enhanced and suitable patient compliance should be the ultimate goal of the prescribing, dispensing, and therapeutic monitoring process. As noted by Sabaté (2003):

> There is not single intervention, strategy or package of strategies that has been shown to be effective across all patients, conditions and settings. Consequently, interventions that target adherence must be tailored to the particular illness-related demands experienced by the patient. To accomplish this, health systems and providers need to develop means of accurately assessing not only adherence, but also those factors that influence it. (p. xiv)

Again, individualization and specificity to patient needs are crucial considerations.

NOTE

1. Medicine-on-Time. http://www.medicine-on-time.com/.

REFERENCES

Blenkinsopp, A., Phelan, M., Bourne, J., & Dakhil, E. (2000). Extended adherence support by community pharmacists for patients with hypertension: A randomized controlled trial. *Int J Pharm Pract, 8:* 165-175.

Bultman, D. C., & Svarstad, B. L. (2000). Effects of physician communication style on client medication beliefs and adherence with antidepressant treatment. *Soc Sci Med, 40:* 173-185.

Carr-Lopez, S. M., Mallett, M. S., & Morse, T. (1995) Tablet splitter: Barrier to compliance or cost-saving instrument? *Am J Health Syst Pharm, 52*(December 1): 2707-2708.

Chisholm, M. A., Mulloy, L. L., Jagadeesan, M., & DiPiro, J. T. (2001). Impact of clinical pharmacy services on renal transplant patients' compliance with immunosuppressive medications. *Clin Transplant, 15:* 330-336.

Cordina, M., McInay, J. C., & Hughes, C. M. (2001). Assessment of a community pharmacy-based program for patients with asthma. *Pharmacotherapy, 21:* 1196-1203.

Dunbar, J. M., Marshall, G. D., & Hovell, M. F. (1979). Behavioral strategies for improving compliance. Chapter 11 in Haynes, R. B., Taylor, D. W., & Sacket, D. L. (Eds.), *Compliance in health care* (pp. 174-190). Baltimore: The Johns Hopkins University Press.

Englehardt, J. B., Allnatt, R., Mariano, A., & Gao, J. (2001). An evaluation of the functionality and acceptability of the voice prescription label. *J Vis Impair Blind, 95*(11): 702-706.

Fincham, J.E. (1998). The drug use process. Chapter 15 in Fincham, J. E., & Wertheimer, A. I. (Eds.), *Pharmacy and the U.S. health care system* (2nd ed.) (pp. 395-438). Binghamton, NY: Haworth Press.

Fincham, J. E., & Wertheimer, A. I. (1985) Using the Health Belief Model to predict initial drug therapy defaulting. *Soc Sci Med, 20*(1): 101-105.

Forcinio, H. (1993). Packaging solutions that help patient compliance. *Pharm. Technol, 17*(March): 44, 46, 48, 50.

Haynes, R. B., McDonald, H. P., & Garg, A. X. (2002). Helping patients follow prescribed treatment applications. *JAMA, 288*(22): 2880-2883.

Hoek, A. J. M. (2003). The role of pharmacists in improving adherence. In Sabaté, E. (Ed.), *Adherence to long-term therapies: Evidence for action* (pp. 159-160). World Health Organization, Geneva, Switzerland.

Hughes, R., & Ortiz, E. (2005). Medication Errors: Why they happen, and how they can be prevented. *American Journal of Nursing, 105*(3): 14-24.

McDonald, H. P., Garg, A. X., & Haynes, R. B. (2002). Interventions to enhance patient adherence to medication prescriptions, Scientific review. *JAMA, 288*(22): 2868-2879.

Perri, M., Martin, B. C., & Pritchard, F. L. (1995). Improving medication compliance: Practical intervention. *J Pharm Technol,* 11(July-August): 167-172.

Peterson, A. M., Takiya, L., & Finley, R. (2003). Meta-analysis of trials of interventions to improve medication adherence. *Am J Health Syst Pharm, 60*(7): 657-665.

Rigby M. (2002). Pharmaceutical packaging can induce confusion. *BMJ, 324:* 679.

Sabaté, E. (Ed.). (2003). *Adherence to long-term therapies: Evidence for action.* World Health Organization, Geneva, Switzerland.

Schulz, M., Verheyen, F., Muhlig, S., Muller, J. M., Muhlbauer, K., Knop-Schneickert, E., Petermann, F., & Bergmann, K. C. (2001). Pharmaceutical care services for asthma patients: A controlled intervention study. *J Clin Pharm, 41:* 668-676.

Segarra, J., DeStefano, J. J., & Davis, R. H. (1991). Streamlining outpatient prescription dispensing utilizing prescriber order entry. ASHP Midyear Clinical Meeting, P-425D, December 26.

Stevenson, F., Barry, C., Britten, N. Barber, N ., & Bradley, C. P . (2000). Doctor-patient communication about drugs: The evidence for shared decision making. *Soc Sci Med, 50:* 829-840.

Thomas, C. P. (2003). Incentive-based formularies. *NEJM, 349*(23): 2186-2187.

Tiano, F. J. (1994). Compliant packaging. *Clin Res Regul Aff, 11*(1): 39-46.

Urquhart, J. (1993). When outpatient drug treatment fails: Identifying noncompliers as a cost-containment tool. *Med Interface,* 6(April): 65-67, 71-73.

Wingender, W., & Kuppers, J. (1993). Bayer compliance device. *Drug Inf J, 27*(4): 1103-1106.

Chapter 8

Bridging the Gap Between Provider and Patient Variables: Concordance

THE CONCORDANCE MOVEMENT IN CONCEPT AND ACTION

The issue of changing the medication-taking paradigm from one of paternalistic control, suggestion, or admonishment to one of a shared process of communicating and agreeing on therapeutic options is a goal for the process of empowering patients to be better compliers. Listed here is a significant body of work and literature related to British efforts to focus on concordance rather than insistance on patient compliance. According to Marinker (2000), concordance can be defined as:

> A new approach to the prescribing and taking of medicines. It is an agreement reached after negotiation between a patient and a health care professional that respects the beliefs and wishes of the patient in determining whether, when and how medicines are to be taken. Although reciprocal, this is an alliance in which the health care professionals recognise the primacy of the patient's decisions about taking the recommended medications. (p. 93)

Shuttleworth (2004) also notes:

> However, to improve concordance, health care professionals need to understand patients' reasons for not taking their medication as prescribed. While in many cases these reasons are relatively straightforward, others are complex and difficult to identify. (p. 29)

Patient Compliance with Medications: Issues and Opportunities
© 2007 by The Haworth Press, Inc. All rights reserved.
doi:10.1300/5365_08

A working party was assigned the task of examining patient compliance and improving on aspects of medication taking by the Royal Pharmaceutical Society of Great Britain in 1995. The task force completed its work with the issuing of a report: From Compliance to Concordance (Royal Pharmaceutical Society, 1997). Elwyn and colleagues (2003) note that there is little evidence at present indicating that the approach leads to better outcomes, but the approach suggests that the involvement of patients in discussions of beliefs about medications, side effects, and harm and benefits being shared will lead to better and safer care.

The use of the term concordance is not new; Hulka and colleagues (1976) researched the relationship of compliance and concordance. Hulka et al. (1976) examined physicians and patients with diabetes mellitus or congestive heart failure. In the context of medication errors due to a lack of concordance between physicians and patients, the researchers determined that there were resultant consequences to the lack of concordance that included four types of medication errors:

- omissions,
- commissions,
- scheduling misconceptions, and
- scheduling noncompliance.

According to Hulka et al. (1976):

> Specific aspects of the medication regimen were associated with increased errors: (1) the more drugs involved between the doctor-patient pair, the greater the errors of omission and commission; and (2) the greater the complexity of the scheduling, the greater the errors of commission and scheduling misconceptions. If the patient did not know the function of all his drugs, errors of commission and scheduling misconception increased. (p. 852)

Hulka and colleagues (1976) focused on doctors' orders and directives—not that this was unimportant, but the definition of concordance has changed as will be seen later. In effect, Maniker (2000, 2004) and colleagues were concerned with respect for the health beliefs of both patient and physician; they did not presume a superiority aspect of physicians' wishes.

Certainly the ramifications of such miscommunication between provider and patient leading to noncompliance have been documented in a large number of studies since this paper by Hulka et al. (1976) was published thirty years ago (Calderon & Beltran, 2004; Chavunduka et al., 1991; Cochrane, Horne, & Chanez, 1999; Davis, 1994; Eldh, Ehnfors, & Eckman, 2004; Fletcher, 1989; Gallagher, 1997; Kjellgren, Ahlner, & Cotter, 1995; Kollaritsch & Wiedermann, 1992; Korver, Goorissen, & Guillebaud, 1995; La Valleur & Wysaocki, 2001; Loghman-Adham, 2003; Lugoboni et al., 2004; McGraw & Drennan, 2001; McPhee & Bird, 1990; Sung, 1999; Weintraub, 1990).

Marinker (2004) notes that the term concordance was in fact first used by Hulka et al. (1976), but that the definitions and concepts involved in concordance go way past what Hulka et al. (1976) described.

Physicians are notoriously poor at predicting their patients' compliance behavior (Becker, 1985). Noble (1998) concludes when considering nonadherence and patients' interactions with physicians:

> The good news is that we now know that non-adherence is not the inexplicable and baffling phenomenon that it was originally considered to be. Both adherence and non-adherence are behaviours can be reliably predicted and one of the key determinants in this is the nature of the communication between the patient and the doctor. (p. 73)

However, even with exquisite models and physicians self-selected for willingness to enhance communication with patients, Stevenson and colleagues (2000) found that key tenets of involvement of both physician and patient and shared decision making did not produce the necessary elements for shared decision making. Shakib and George (2003) suggest that bad prescribing frequently involves writing a prescription for a symptom or a diagnosis and not considering the other steps in the prescribing process. They suggest that therapeutic goals are the answer to the patient's question: "Why am I taking this medication?" They continue: "Taking this step in the prescribing process allows for a greater consideration of available treatment options, greater individualisation of therapy, avoids treatment on the basis of surrogate endpoints, and may result in greater patient concordance" (p. 147).

Education, reinforcement, and a shift from paternalistic views of the patient will be necessary ingredients to move forward with a shared approach to patient care and decision making.

Specific Disease States

Chapman and colleagues (2000) note that for asthmatics, doctors need to use a range of communication skills and approaches that respect individual health beliefs as a tool to improve doctor–patient interactions. Chapman and colleagues (2000) suggest these actions: ". . . can help to foster an atmosphere of mutual responsibility and concordance" (p. 9).

Gray and colleagues (2002), when reviewing the literature pertinent to antipsychotic behavior, note that increasing education influences understanding of diseases, but not necessarily better compliance behavior. They suggest that compliance therapy, based on cognitive-behavioral techniques, appear to be effective in enhancing compliance and preventing relapse (Gray, Wykes, & Gpurnay, 2002). Hull and colleagues (2005) suggest that less reliance on a biomedical paradigm and more on behavioral strategies may explain differences in treatment success of patients taking antidepressant medications, such as selective serotonin reuptake inhibitors (SSRIs).

Pollock and Grime (2000) note that patients who were prescribed proton pump inhibitors (PPIs) can self-regulate consumption of the drugs this can "lead to an overall reduction in PPI prescribing and associated costs, and an increase in patient autonomy and control which is in line with the concordance model of the ideal relationship between patients and doctors" (p. 1827).

Patients with Special Needs—Seniors

Due to the increasing morbidity associated with seniors and subsequent drug compliance issues, authors, when speaking of concordance, mention that reductions in the quantity of drugs prescribed and prescribers' use of standard prescribing indicators are tools to consider to improve seniors' concordance with medication therapies

(Banning, 2004). Banning (2004) also suggests that education be an integral part of patient care and not just a portion of discharge activities. Further, it is suggested that both verbal and written counseling that is patient centered can help seniors to more appropriately solve medication mismanagement problems.

When considering aspirin therapy and stroke patients, Short and colleagues (2003) posit that noncompliance in prescribing aspirin treatment for stroke patients may in fact either be noncompliance, a lack of following a prescribing guideline, or in fact may be concordance between patients and physicians choosing a nonaspirin option as treatment. They note: "It is not possible to assess whether low levels of prescribing reflect appropriate or inappropriate use of aspirin in specific patients where concordance between the GP and the patient is practiced" (p. 9).

Pediatric Patients

Costello and colleagues (2004), when conducting a review of the literature pertaining to medication use in children, note that concordance, compliance, and medicines access by pediatric patients show lower rates of compliance than that associated with older age groups. As children approach adolescence, rebellious behavior may further diminish compliance activities. The authors suggest a comprehensive approach including school-based medicines education and outreach clinics as a method to improve pediatric patient drug-taking patterns (Costello, Wong, & Nunn, 2004). Several countries, most notably Scotland, have incorporated medication teaching into grammar school curricula (Learning and Teaching Scotland, 2000). This teaching of the importance and relevance of proper medication use will no doubt pay dividends as youngsters matriculate through the educational system and become better and more informed medicine-taking patients.

CONCORDANCE

Following the recommendations of working groups dealing with concordance, the then Junior Health Minister in the United Kingdom, Lord P. Hunt set in place funding for the Medicines Partnership (www

.medicine-partnership.org). According to the Web site of The Task Force on Medicines Partnership,

> The Task Force on Medicines Partnership is a Department of Health funded program which aims to help patients to get the most out of medications, by involving them as partners in prescribing decisions and supporting them in medicine taking. The program was announced by Lord Hunt in April 2001 and formally established in January 2002 with £1.3m of funding from the Pharmacy in the Future project to cover a work program of two years (2002 and 2003). Funding for a second phase through to summer 2005 was confirmed at the start of 2004.[1]

As can be seen in Figure 8.1, there are three pillars with four components totally making up concordance. These four requirements are as follows:

1. Patients have enough knowledge to participate as partners.
2. Health professionals are prepared for partnership.
3. Prescribing consultations involve patients as partners.
4. Patients are supported in taking medicines.

As can be seen, key tenets in the concordance model include empowerment of patients, investiture of time and assistance by caregivers, a sense of involvement on the part of patients, shared and informed decision making, and feedback and restructuring input, and use of medications over time. A crucial component of concordance is the placing of patients' health beliefs center stage in the joint decision-making approach used by patients and physicians and other health providers (Horne & Weinman, 2004). Tones (1998) suggests that health promotion and focusing on the patient proactively averts the blame-the-victim approach so common in the past when examining patient adherence.

Shaw (2004a) has outlined three constituent elements that are needed for implementation:

1. patients have access to the information, knowledge and skills they need to participate as partners in prescribing decisions,
2. prescribing consultations involving patients as partners in shared decisions about treatment,

3. patients supported in taking their medication according to the concordant agreement that has been made. (p. 148)

Shaw (2004b) also notes that interventions must be patient tailored to meet patient needs; simple provision of information or materials without a probing and considering of the patient's perspective is fraught with difficulties.

There is not a single model or approach that will meet all the needs of all patients and providers. Concordance in and of itself is not the perfect model to be emulated by all. What it does is bring a fresh and much-needed change in perspective on how to impact patient non-compliance in a fluid series of implemented steps. Now it is up to re-

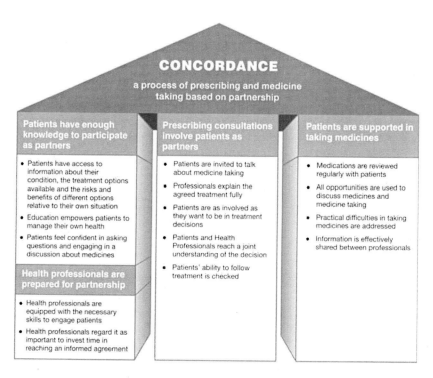

FIGURE 8.1. Concordance. (*Souce:* "What Is Concordance" www.medicines-partnership.org/about-us/concordance. Reprinted with permission from Medicines Partnership, London, U.K.)

searchers and practitioners to implement and evaluate programs that
have incorporated the fresh new approach of concordance.

NOTE

1. http//:www.medicine-partnership.org.

REFERENCES

Banning, M. (2004). Enhancing older people's concordance with taking their medication. *Br J Nurs, 13*(11): 669-674.

Becker, M. H. (1985). Patient adherence to prescribed therapies. *Medical Care, 23:*
539-555.

Calderon, J. L. & Beltran, R. A. (2004). Pitfalls in health communication: Healthcare policy, institution, structure, and process. *MedGenMed, 6*(1): 9.

Chapman, K. R., Walker, L., Cluley, S., & Fabbri, L. (2000). Improving patient compliance with asthma therapy. *Respir Med, 94*(1): 2-9.

Chavunduka, D., Dzimwasha, M., Madondo, F., Mafana, E., Mbewe, A., & Nyazema,
N. Z. (1991). Drug information for patients in the community. *World Health
Forum, 12*(1): 29-33.

Cochrane, G. M., Horne, R., & Chanez, P. (1999). Compliance in asthma. *Respir
Med, 93*(11): 763-769.

Costello, I., Wong, I. C., & Nunn, A. J. (2004). A literature review to identify interventions to improve the use of medicines in children. *Child Care Health Dev,
30*(6): 647-665.

Davis, A. J. (1994). The role of hormonal contraception in adolescents. *Am J Obstet
Gynecol, 170*(5 Pt 2): 1581-1585.

Eldh, A. C., Ehnfors, M., & Eckman, I. (2004). The phenomena of participation and
non-participation in health care—experiences of patients attending a nurse-led
clinic for chronic heart failure. *Eur J Cardiovasc Nurs, 3*(3): 239-246.

Elwyn, G., A. Edwards, & Britten, N. (2003). "Doing prescribing": How might clinicians work differently for better, safer care. *Qual Saf Health Care, 12*(Suppl 1):
i33-i36.

Fletcher, R. H. (1989). Patient compliance with therapeutic advice: A modern view.
Mt Sinai J Med, 56(6): 453-458.

Gallagher, S. M. (1997). Powerlessness as a factor in health defeating behavior.
Ostomy Wound Manage, 43(2): 34-36, 38, 40, 42.

Gray, R., Wykes, T., & Gpurnay, K. (2002). From compliance to concordance: A review of the literature on interventions to enhance compliance with antipsychotic
medication. *J Psychiatr Ment Health Nurs, 9*(3): 277-284.

Horne, R. & Weinman, J. (2004). The theoretical basis of concordance and issues
for research. Chapter 7 in Bond, Christine (Ed.), *Concordance* (p. 142). London:
The Pharmaceutical Press, RPSGB.

Hulka, B. S., Cassel, J. C., Kupper, L., & Burdette, J. (1976). Communication, compliance, and concordance between physicians and patients with prescribed medications. *Am J Public Health, 66*(9): 847-853.

Hull, S. A., Aquino, P., & Cotter, S. (2005). Explaining variation in antidepressant prescribing rates in east London: A cross sectional study. *Fam Pract, 22*(1): 37-42.

Kjellgren, K. I., Ahlner, J., & Cotter, S. (1995) Taking antihypertensive medication—controlling or co-operating with patients? *Int J Cardiol, 47*(3): 257-268.

Kollaritsch, H., & G. Wiedermann (1992). Compliance of Austrian tourists with prophylactic measures. *Eur J Epidemiol, 8*(2): 243-251.

Korver, T., Goorissen, E., & Guillebaud, J. (1995). The combined oral contraceptive pill: What advice should we give when tablets are missed? *Br J Obstet Gynaecol, 102*(8): 601-607.

La Valleur, J., & Wysocki, S. (2001). Selection of oral contraceptives or hormone replacement therapy: Patient communication and counseling issues. *Am J Obstet Gynecol, 185*(2 Suppl): S57-64.

Learning and Teaching Scotland. (2000). *Health education guide for teachers and managers.* Glasgow, Scotland, UK: Learning and Teaching Scotland.

Loghman-Adham, M. (2003). Medication noncompliance in patients with chronic disease: Issues in dialysis and renal transplantation. *Am J Manag Care, 9*(2): 155-171.

Lugoboni, F., Quaglio, G., Mezzelani, P., Pajusco, B., Casari, R., & Lechi, A. (2004). Improving compliance in internal medicine: The motivational discussion. *Ann Ital Med Int, 19*(3): 155-162.

Marinker, M. (2000). Achieving concordance. *Primary Care Pharmacy,* September, *1*(4): 93-95.

Marinker M. (2004). From compliance to concordance: A personal view. Chapter 1 in Bond, Christine (Ed.), *Concordance* (p. 5). London: The Pharmaceutical Press, RPSGB.

McGraw, C. & Drennan, V. (2001). Self-administration of medicine and older people. *Nurs Stand, 15*(18): 33-36.

McPhee, S. J. & Bird, J. A. (1990). Implementation of cancer prevention guidelines in clinical practice. *J Gen Intern Med, 5*(5 Suppl): S116-122.

Noble, L. M. (1998). Doctor-patient communication and adherence to treatment. Chapter 3 in Myers, L. B. & Midence, K. (Eds.), *Adherence to treatment in medical conditions* (pp. 51-82). UK: Harwood Academic Publishers.

Pollock, K. & Grime, J. (2000). Strategies for reducing the prescribing of proton pump inhibitors (PPIs): Patient self-regulation of treatment may be an underexploited resource. *Soc Sci Med, 51*(12): 1827-1839.

Royal Pharmaceutical Society of Great Britain (1997). *From compliance to concordance. Achieving shared goals in medicine taking.* London: Royal Pharmaceutical Society of Great Britain.

Shaw, J. (2004a). A policy framework for concordance. Chapter 8 in Bond, Christine (Ed.), *Concordance* (p. 148). London: The Pharmaceutical Press, RPSGB.

Shaw, J. (2004b). A policy framework for concordance. Chapter 8 in Bond, Christine (Ed.), *Concordance* (p. 162). London: The Pharmaceutical Press, RPSGB.

Shakib, S. & George, A. (2003). Diagnosis and therapeutic goals. What are you actually treating? *Aust Fam Physician, 32*(3): 147-149.

Short, D., Frischer, M., Bashford, J., & Ashcroft, D. (2003). Why are eligible patients not prescribed aspirin in primary care? A qualitative study indicating measures for improvement. *BMC Fam Pract, 4*(1): 9.

Shuttleworth, A. (2004). Improving drug concordance in patients with chronic conditions. *Nurs Times, 100*(24): 28-29.

Stevenson, F. A., Barry, C. A., Britten, N., Barber, N., & Bradley, C. P. (2000). Doctor-patient communication about drugs: The evidence for shared decision making. *Social Science & Medicine, 50:* 829-840.

Sung, C. L. (1999). Asian Patients' distrust of western medical care: One perspective. *Mt Sinai J Med, 66*(4): 259-261.

Tones, K. (1998). Health promotion: Empowering choice. Chapter 6 in Myers, L. B., & Midence, K. (Eds.), *Adherence to treatment in medical conditions* (pp. 133-160). UK: Harwood Academic Publishers.

Weintraub, M. (1990). Compliance in the elderly. *Clin Geriatr Med, 6*(2): 445-452.

Chapter 9

Ethics of Compliance

This chapter focuses on the ethical issues surrounding compliance for some patients and on the ethics of forcing someone to be compliant. There are instances when the complex issues surrounding compliance become even more complex, and ethical issues may override therapeutics and decision making (Jonsen, 1980). Self-medication, paternalism, assisted suicide, death by lethal injection, Plan B emergency contraception, or even pharmacists' refusal of filling of oral contraceptive prescriptions place the focus on the ethics of decision making. These decisions are made by practitioners (physicians, nurses, pharmacists, family members, caregivers, correctional facility personnel, and/or individual patients). Pharmaceutical manufacturers evoke ethical concerns when drugs are put on the market based upon assumptions that data derived from clinical trials were assumed to have emanated from compliant patients from the varying groups compared during studies. Individuals would do well to consider how they will respond to ethical considerations in varying decision-making situations.

Is it reasonable to conclude that in the interest of the greater good it is acceptable to coerce an incompetent individual to be compliant? When evaluating competency of an individual, an assessment of decision-making capacity is the accepted procedure for determining when a person is not competent. This can be a murky area. Silberfeld and Checkland (1999) note such in the following: "An inferential gap exists between the criteria for capacity specific abilities and the legal requirements to understand relevant information and appreciate the consequences of a decision" (p. 377).

Patient Compliance with Medications: Issues and Opportunities
© 2007 by The Haworth Press, Inc. All rights reserved.
doi:10.1300/5365_09

They go on to suggest that a multidisciplinary approach is appropriate in the process of determining competence.

When patients are noncompliant with regimens due to lack of resources for payment, should they receive less care than others due to their economically driven noncompliance? What should happen after refusal to comply? should fewer health resources be provided for these individuals (Savulescu, 1998)? How about the right of refusal to take medications (Howe, 1988)? More often than not the ethics of compliance and coercion relate to the use of psychotropic medications in subpopulations (Beighley & Brown, 1992; Rosenson, 1993). Psychogeriatric patients pose a special patient population at risk due to increased vulnerability associated with aging patients (Wood, 1986). Wood (1986) notes that elderly depressed patients may not cooperate with caregivers due to fear of loss of independence, impaired cognition, and reasoning ability, perhaps sabotaged by others, or a bias toward treatment due to unfair stereotyping of mental disorders and treatment. Social workers, more than any other health professional group, struggle with the ethics of compliance by mental health patients and coercion (Bentley, 1993; Rosenson, 1993; Wilk, 1994).

Tuberculosis (TB) patients present a classic patient population where ethics and the public good can clash relative to coercive treatment requirements (Reilly, 1993). When do individual rights need to surpass or be subservient to the health rights of others? Is it fair to be exposed to horrible infectious diseases, which in some cases may be resistant to therapy, in order to hold an individual who is noncompliant harmless for being nonadherent. Unchecked tuberculosis, or undertreated TB, affects those without the ability to make informed decisions, for example, the newborn (Guthrie, 2005).

CAPITAL PUNISHMENT
AND ASSISTED SUICIDE

Two circumstances of compliance with medications lead to intentional mortality. Here compliance takes on an understandably different aspect. When drugs are administered, either by lethal injection in a prison or self-administered to achieve death by suicide, compliance leads to purposeful negative consequences. Psychological ramifications for those who prescribe, dispense, administer, or otherwise approve of such use of medications may follow these decisions made to consciously end a human life.

NONCOMPLIANCE
AS A PATIENT PREROGATIVE

Patients are noncompliant purposely in many settings, including hospitals where administration of medications is routine (Canada & Lesko, 1980). In the ambulatory setting, noncompliance can be on purpose or it can be incidental (Johnson, Williams, & Marshal, 1999). Patients may make such noncompliant decisions based upon many factors that may include their individual health beliefs, lack of faith in prescribers or therapy prescribed, occurrence of adverse drug reactions, or depression due to the realization of the need for a long-term therapy.

Hughes (2004) takes the view that patient noncompliance by seniors may in fact be "intelligent noncompliance" to avoid adverse effects or lack of therapeutic benefit. In some cases by self-monitoring of conditions or symptoms, patients may feel that it may not be necessary for them to continue to take medications. Some drugs are prescribed on an as-needed basis. Examples here might be oral antihistamines for allergies that may vary during the year, and may not need to be taken year round. In another instance, the dose of a drug such as insulin to treat diabetes may require an alteration in the amount injected, or a decision whether it is to be taken via an insulin pump.

Another factor leading to noncompliance with seniors, or other patients for that matter, is economically driven. Although the cost aspect of noncompliance has been mentioned earlier in the book, it is worth repeating here in the context of ethics associated with economic noncompliance. Ethics relate to manufacturers' profit-driven ethos, driving patients to be noncompliant due to the high cost of pharmacotherapy.

Also, a patient may need to alter how they take a drug such as digoxin (Lanoxin) to treat congestive heart failure if their pulse falls below a certain minimum amount. Other drugs such as sodium warfarin (Coumadin) may require that the dose be changed from time to time and require patients to be intelligently noncompliant. The dosing of many drugs is more "art" than "science" and may require that patients be intelligently noncompliant with prescribed therapies.

HEALTH INSURANCE PORTABILITY AND ACCOUNTABILITY (HIPPA) ACT AND IMPACTS UPON COMPLIANCE

In 1996, the U.S. Congress recognized the need for national patient record privacy standards by enacting a legislative act entitled the Health Insurance Portability and Accountability Act of 1996 (HIPAA). The law was enacted to protect private health information (PHI), as well as to provide for other matters. PHI relates to the physical or mental health of an individual, the provision of health care to an individual, or the payment for health care for an individual and identifies the individual, or it can be used to identify the individual.

The law specified provisions designed to save money for health care entities by encouraging electronic transactions, but it also required new safeguards to protect the security and confidentiality of patient health care information. As is apparent when receiving any type of health care services in the past few years, patients are presented with a detailed description of these requirements, are asked (or have been asked) to sign that they have been provided the information, and are provided a copy of the HIPAA regulations as they pertain to the specific care that a patient is receiving. Regarding prescription medications, others, beside the patient, cannot access the records of other family members; however, they can pick up prescriptions for other family members (children, spouses, parents, etc.).

U.S. Federal Law provides the right to patients to:

1. request that restrictions be placed on certain uses and disclosures of health information,
2. know that individuals can inspect their medical records, and
3. know that they can obtain copies of their medical records.

Let me just say a word or two about medical records. Patients have a record of care throughout the many places that they receive health care services. Thus, every time they see a physician, are hospitalized, or fill a prescription, a record of this activity is updated at each respective point of receiving care. Although patients' health records are the physical property of the health care practitioner (or institution; pharmacy, laboratory, allied health professional) that has compiled it, the information itself belongs to patients.

Physicians must allow patients to view their medical records, even if they have not paid their bill (Mulder, 2004). Physicians may request that this request be put in writing, and perhaps even require patients to have such letters notarized. When you do request information from your medical records, be as specific as possible.

Patient compliance interventions must be made with the consent of the patient. Patients must explicitly do so. Before patients can be placed on mailing lists of any sort related to medication compliance, they must specifically approve of placement on a mailing list that is related to the care that they are receiving. It is not uncommon at present in the United States for pharmacies to be contacted by manufacturers to be able to contact patients encouraging the filling or refilling of prescriptions. These letters and mass mail attempts to encourage compliance are notoriously ineffective. Often the information contained in the letter is erroneous, outdated, or dated in scope and content. Many times the prescription may have already been filled, refilled, or perhaps discontinued on the request of the physician before the patient receives it. The FDA-approved professional package insert is often included in the mailing, which is a telltale sign that a pharmaceutical manufacturer is behind the ineffective ploy.

Before being placed on such mailing lists, due to HIPPA regulations, patients must consent for providers and/or manufacturers to contact them in this manner. If patients specifically request to have their name withdrawn from such lists, this request is required to be complied with by all involved. Even in an age of emerging electronic medical records potential and synergy, consumers are being encouraged to rigorously protect their health information and access as they protect financial, credit, or other important information sources.

The U.S. government defines PHI (U.S. National Institutes of Health, 2005) as

individually identifiable health information, held or maintained by a covered entity or its business associates acting for the covered entity, that is transmitted or maintained in any form or medium (including the individually identifiable health information of non-U.S. citizens). This includes identifiable demographic and other information relating to the past, present, or future physical or mental health or condition of an individual, or the provision or payment of health care to an individual that is created or received by a health care provider, health plan, employer, or health care clearinghouse. For purposes of the Privacy Rule, genetic information is considered to be health information.

If patients are receiving care in a hospital or in another health care institution (e.g., long-term care facility, independent living facility), there are institutional review boards (IRBs) that monitor the care provided, including the drugs that may be prescribed. If by chance, patients are taking an investigational drug, an IRB had to provide approval for the manufacturer or investigators to administer or provide the drug to patients. Efforts to encourage compliance in such instances through varying compliance interventions must also be approved by the IRB. To do so without IRB approval is certainly unethical and illegal.

The HIPAA Act was passed to do a number of things including making it easier for employees to retain health coverage after leaving an employer. HIPPA regulations also provided for increased overseeing of cases of health care fraud and abuse. In the decade of the 1990s, the tracking of abuse and fraud in the health care system increased dramatically due to HIPPA provisions (Steinhauer, 2001).

INFORMATION TECHNOLOGY

Currently, we live in an age of information technology eclipsing our ability to properly monitor what is being transmitted and to whom. Unless safeguards are in place this transfer of information can have not only positive but negative consequences. Computerization of medical and pharmacy records affords providers and institutions unique ways to store voluminous amounts of health data with little or no expansive storage necessary as was the case in the past. Compliance interventions can be developed with technology available; however, important safeguards need to be in place to ensure that only those who should see health data see it.

Organizations should develop clear-cut, explicit policies to monitor security and confidentiality of computerized medical records and records of compliance interventions (Committee on Maintaining Privacy and Security in Health Care Applications of the National Information Infrastructure, 1997). You should be able to review audit logs of accesses to your medical records. Ethical lapses occur, and therefore resultant incidents, and when this happens, it is hard to imagine how it could have happened. For example, in April 2004, prescription records at the University of Kansas Student Health Center were possibly accessed by a computer hacker (Weslander, 2004). This affected thousands of students, faculty, and staff members' records at KU. Officials still do not know who did it and how it happened. This is inexcusable in this day and time. So, it is important to ensure that these types of lapses, which may include the transmission of pertinent information regarding patient compliance, do not occur.

When records are hacked, information gleaned could reveal credit card information, sensitive health information, or personal information that is sensitive in nature. This is not an inconsequential happening—it is serious, and patients have legal recourse should it happen.

QUESTIONABLE, IF NOT, UNETHICAL PRACTICES

Several pharmaceutical company issues may be perceived in a very negative light. These include direct-to-consumer advertising, educational programs, and the naming of drugs themselves. Medication misuse and noncompliance can be the negative result of both how drugs are named and how they are advertised.

Drug-Company-Supplied Patient Leaflets

In the guise of patient education and provision of written information, some pharmaceutical companies and pharmacies engage in confusing practices regarding patient leaflets that accompany new and refill prescriptions when dispensed. Although intentions may be good, patient outcomes may be poor. An example of such confusion can be found when leaflets are customized to provide some information about the drug. For example, one side of the leaflet may provide information pertaining to the drug: how to take the drug and some common side effects and other warnings. The other side of the leaflet may list information for another drug also used to treat the illness. Unless the patients are savvy enough to realize the drug information on the right is being advertised by a competitor drug and the drug information listed on the left is information about the drug dispensed they may become very confused. Sometimes, the amount of the material pertinent to the drug not dispensed, yet advertised on the leaflet, is much greater in scope and depth than the scant information provided for the actual drug dispensed. This type of educational leaflet is extremely objectionable. To further compound the potential for error, the dispensing pharmacist may or may not counsel the patient on the drug being dispensed, and provide supplementary information about the actual drug prescribed for the patient. This type of direct-to-consumer advertising is misguided. Is the patient to think the drug dispensed is less preferred? Do they feel inadequate that they did not receive the drug on the right?

Or do they realize the drug information specific for ezetimibe that is listed is not for the drug they have been prescribed, and are noncompliant because of confusion?

Confusing Drug Names

The naming of drugs is confusing for practitioners and can certainly be for patients as well. Confusing names lead to medication errors and noncompliance as well. Confused patients are less likely to be compliant than other patients (Feinberg, Tobias, & Cameron, 2000). Drug-name confusion starts with the naming of drugs and similarity with other drugs on the market. Rados (2005), when writing of drug-name confusion and medication errors notes: "Drug companies want a name that will boost sales, while consumers long for some indication of what the drug does" (p. 45).

A light-hearted look at drug names and where they come from can be found in Figure 9.1. With some of the confusing names that are present it is curious where the names of drugs do in fact come from. The U.S. FDA indicates that approximately 10 percent of drug errors

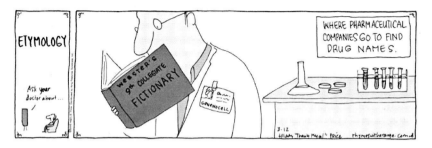

FIGURE 9.1. Rhymes with Orange. (*Source:* © Hilary B. Price. Reprinted with special permission of King Features Syndicate.)

are due to confusion regarding the names of drugs. Errors of omission by pharmacists and physicians occur when computerized listings of drugs become commonplace (Rados, 2005).

PHARMACEUTICAL COMPANY RESEARCH AND CLINICAL TRIALS

Drugs reach the marketplace with profiles detailing the following:

- Dosage
- Pharmacokinetics
- Adverse effects or adverse drug reactions
- Outcomes
- Clinical
- Economic
- Humanistic[1]
- Elimination half-life
- Efficacy rates in comparison with placebo or gold standards achieved in randomized clinical trials (RCTs)

However, prerelease compliance is not an assessment that is measured. Most clinical trials of new pharmaceutical products proceed with the assumption that patients are compliant with the investigational drug, but this is taken for granted rather than empirically tested (Spilker, 1991). The process can be difficult and might be easier to ignore (Goetghebeur & Shipiro, 1996; Pocock & Abdalla, 1998), but it should not be ignored. Arras (1990) notes that HIV patients in AIDS research may refuse treatment with a "coercion defense." However, community involvement and social policies encouraging cooperation can help patients through this process. Proper attention to design issues and full disclosure are crucial for participants to tie in (Schuklenk & Hogan, 1997).

The elderly use three times as many drugs as younger patients, yet this number may actually be understated in seniors due to their lack of economic ability to be compliant (Pavlovich-Danis, 2004). Medications for chronic conditions such as hypertension or dyslipidemia may be under-complied with due to the high cost of therapies (Cunningham, 2002). Seniors face difficulty with economic compliance for several reasons; a recent Henry J. Kaiser Family Foundation publication (2005) examining drugs use and the elderly determined the following:

- 73 percent of seniors take five or more prescription medications,
- 57 percent take more than one type of prescription,
- 67 percent utilize more than one prescribing physician, and
- 41 percent utilize more than one pharmacy. (p. 45)

In the same report (Henry J. Kaiser Family Foundation, 2005), it was noted that 52 percent of seniors with three or more chronic conditions are noncompliant (p. 45). Again with those seniors with three or more chronic conditions:

- 35 percent skipped, took smaller doses, or did not initially fill prescriptions because of cost,
- 19 percent did not fill prescriptions because they thought the drug was not necessary. (p. 45)

This is a crucial issue for seniors, and the Medicare Part D prescription drug benefit, although projected to help some seniors in some way, will not address the issue of drug company charges for prescription drugs. The enabling legislation was passed with the provision that CMS personnel could not negotiate prices with the pharmaceutical manufacturers.

In summary, differing levels of ethical considerations and varying strata of severity/intensity/ramifications are significant influences on patient compliance. This aspect of compliance affects each of us, certainly in many different ways. But nonetheless, it is vital that all involved in drug taking and compliance issues realize the individual ethical consideration as well as the ethical ramification on others. The resultant decisions that people choose to make need to be carefully considered and understood by stakeholders in patient compliance or lack thereof.

NOTE

1. Sociobehavioral components that may include quality of life, patient satisfaction, well-being (self-assessed, and not provider assessed), etc.

REFERENCES

Arras, J. D. (1990). Noncompliance in AIDS research. *Hastings Cent Rep, 20*(5): 24-32.

Beighley, P. S., & Brown, G. R. (1992). Medication refusal by psychiatric inpatients in the military. *Milit Med, 157*(1): 47-49.

Bentley, K. J. (1993). The right of psychiatric patients to refuse medications: Where should social workers stand? *Soc Work, 38*(1): 101-106.

Canada, A. T., & Lesko, L. J. (1980). Two reasons for unusual therapeutic drug monitoring results in hospitalized patients. *Ther Drug Monit, 2*(3): 217-219.

Committee on Maintaining Privacy and Security in Health Care Applications of the National Information Infrastructure. (1997). For the record, protecting electronic health information. Washington, DC: National Academy Press.

Cunningham, P. J. (2002). Prescription drug access: Not just a Medicare problem. Issue Brief from HSC, *51*(2):1-4, Washington, DC: Center for Studying Health System Change.

Feinberg, J. L., Tobias, D. E., & Cameron, K. A. (2000). MDS-Med Guide: Assessing medication effects using patient assessment data. *AACP-Annual-Meeting* (American-Association-of-Colleges-of-Pharmacy-Annual-Meeting), *101* (July): 49.

Goetghebeur, E., & Shipiro, S. H. (1996). Analyzing non-compliance in clinical trials: Ethical imperative or mission impossible. *Stat Med, 15:* 2813-2826.

Guthrie, P. TB warning from hospital brings flood of request for tests. *The Atlanta Journal Constitution,* July 20, 2005. http://www.ajc.com/news/content/metro/northfulton/0705/20northside.html. Accessed July 22, 2005.

Henry, J. Kaiser Family Foundation (2005). *Medicare Chartbook* (3rd ed) (Summer), Washington, DC.

Howe, E. G. (1988). Ethical aspects of geriatric patients' rights to refuse treatment and to receive limited medical resources. *Educ Gerontol, 14*(5): 451-463. http://privacyruleandresearch.nih.gov/pr_07.asp. Accessed July 23, 2005.

Hughes, C. M. (2004). Medication non-adherence in the elderly: How big is the problem? *Drugs Aging, 21*(12): 793-811.

Johnson, M. J., Williams, M., & Marshal, F. S. (1999). Adherent and nonadherent medication-taking in elderly hypertensive patients. *Clin Nurs Res, 8*(4): 318-335.

Jonsen, A. R. (1980). Ethical meaning of medication. *Art Med* (September) *1*(1): 11-17.

Mulder, J. (August 23, 2004) Request medical records in writing. *Syracuse Post-Standard, Moneywise Health Care Notebook.*

Pavlovich-Danis, S. J. (2004). Differentiating between inability to afford prescription medications and "noncompliance." *Geriat Times,* (May/June) (3): 1-7.

Pocock, S., & Adballa, M. (1998). The hope and hazards of using compliance data in clinical trials. *Stat Mede, 17:* 303-317.

Rados, D. (2005) Drug name confusion: Preventing medication errors. FDA Consumer July/August: 35-37.

Reilly, R. G. (1993). Combating the tuberculosis epidemic: The legality of coercive treatment measures. *Columbia J Law Soc Probl, 27:* 101-149.

Rosenson, M. K. (1993). Social work and the right of psychiatric patients to refuse medication: A family advocate's response. *Soc Work, 38*(1): 107-112.

Savulescu, J. (1998). The cost of refusing treatment and equality of outcome. *J Med Ethics, 24*(4): 231-236.

Schuklenk, U., & Hogan, C. (1997). AIDS clinical trials: Ethical and design issues. *J Int Bioethique, 8*(3): 127-132.

Silberfeld, M., & Checkland, D. (1999). Faulty judgment, expert opinion, and decision-making capacity. *Theor Med Bioeth, 20*(4): 377-393.

Spilker, B. A. (1991). Methods of assessing and improving patient compliance in clinical trials. Chapter 5 in Cramer, J. A., & Spilker, B. (Eds.) *Patient compliance in medical practice and clinical trials* (pp. 37-56). New York: Raven Press, Ltd.

Steinhauer, J. (January 23, 2001). Justice department finds success chasing health care fraud. *The New York Times,* p. A19.

Weslander, E. Website helps prevent ID theft. *Lawrence Journal World,* August 14, 2004.

Wilk, R. J. (1994). Are the rights of people with mental illness still important? *Soc Work, 39*(2): 167-175.

Wood, A. (1986). Uncooperative behavior in unipolar depression: Managing medication non-compliance. Chapter 12 in Brink, T. L. (Ed.), *The elderly uncooperative patient* (pp. 109-122). London: The Haworth Press.

Chapter 10

The Role of Health Professionals
in Influencing Patient Compliance

Richard Schulz

The oath taken by health professionals requires them to dedicate their professional lives to the service of their patients. Congruent with this service is the commitment to act in the best interest of patients in ways that improve the chance of positive health outcomes. Patient compliance with medical advice is viewed as a vital, multifaceted aspect of this care which can influence their well-being. While the scope of noncompliance (Chapter 2 by Jack E. Fincham) and its associated costs (Chapter 3 by Jayashree Shankaranarayanan) are important considerations, the soundest justification for understanding the reason people take or do not take medicines resides in our professional and moral responsibilities to our patients.

Health professionals participate in and influence patients' medication therapy practice in a variety of ways. Chapter 7 by Jack E. Fincham has examined the methods to impact patient compliance. Prior to that, Chapter 6 by Christopher Cook presented and contrasted the models that provide a conceptual framework for those interventions. This chapter focuses on the responsibilities of health professionals as they attempt to move patients to positive health outcomes within the context of the patients' medication practice. Included in these responsibilities are the following: (1) recognize your limitations and bias, (2) make sense of a vast and contradictory literature

Patient Compliance with Medications: Issues and Opportunities
© 2007 by The Haworth Press, Inc. All rights reserved.
doi:10.1300/5365_10

so that relevant information regarding compliance can be processed efficiently, (3) commit to the development of best practices for medication compliance. The chapter concludes with a synthesis of recent trends in the compliance literature and the role of health professionals.

RECOGNIZE LIMITATIONS AND BIASES

Identifying Noncompliant Patients

Health providers, by virtue of their clinical knowledge, communication skills, and presence as a support factor, can influence patients' efforts to comply with medical advice. Furthermore, providers develop and implement strategies to maintain and/or improve compliance among their patients. A reasonable first step in the process would be to recognize the presence of a compliance problem, that is, knowledge might not be imparted, empathy might not be communicated, support might not be offered, and program might not be implemented if the physician, nurse, pharmacist, social worker, and others believe that their patients are following medical advice. Unless the clinician is able to detect and recognize patients' difficulty with following a prescribed regimen, he or she will interpret poor clinical response as a failure of the therapy, instead of a problem of compliance. The reaction would be one of the following: (1) increasing the dose of the prescribed therapy, thereby increasing the risk of side effect or toxicity; (2) augmenting therapy with another drug that brings its own risks, and complicates the existing therapy, making it more likely that the patient will be noncompliant; or (3) discontinuation of the existing medicine, thereby losing the benefit of what was considered the first choice therapy. None of these options is good for the patient and will increase the likelihood of poor outcomes. Clearly, it is in the best interest of the patient and health professional to be able to detect noncompliance.

Chapter 5 by Jack E. Fincham offers a full discussion of the ways of measuring compliance. In our rush to define and measure this behavior, we, by default, trust in our ability to recognize it in our patients. Unfortunately, the literature does not support this contention. Miller et al. (2002) quantified clinicians' ability to identify compliance with antiretroviral therapy. The authors asked physicians, nurse practitioners, residents, and fellows to estimate the percentage of antiretroviral medication taken by their patients over the four weeks preceding the clinical visit, and predictively over the next four weeks. Compliance was assessed using the Medication Event Monitoring System (MEMS), and was calculated as the number of doses taken per day divided by the number of doses prescribed summed over a four-week period and expressed as a percentage. Alternative measures were in place if MEMS data proved unreliable. Clinicians were asked to estimate the percentage of time this patient took the antiretroviral medicine as prescribed. Two measures of compliance were reported: (1) adherence difference and (2) absolute adherence difference. The adherence difference is the clinician's estimate of adherence minus the measured adherence. The absolute adherence difference is the absolute values for both the four weeks before and the predicted upcoming four weeks summed. Mean adherence difference was 8.9 percent. Mean absolute adherence difference was 15.7 percent. For both measures, clinicians overestimated medication adherence, that is, they believed their patients were more adherent with prescribed regimen than they actually were. Adherence difference was greater than 10 percent in 35 percent of cases, and greater than 20 percent in 21 percent of cases. Sensitivity was 24 to 62 percent, indicating that the clinicians were not able to identify many nonadherent patients. The authors concluded that clinicians' inability to identify nonadherence in their patients represent missed opportunities to intervene and improve adherence.

Relying on one's intuition or preconceived notions about who might be noncompliant is ineffective and inefficient. Health professionals can improve their ability to identify noncompliant patients by utilizing the literature that identifies factors associated with compliance. As discussed later in the chapter, these can be patient factors, social and economic factors, condition-related factors, therapy or treatment factors, and health care team and system-related factors. The second avenue for health providers is to engage in an ongoing dialogue with patients regarding the meaning of medicine to them. Open-ended questions that allow patients to tell their story will yield the necessary information to inform clinicians about patient's medication-taking behavior.

The Extent of Our Influence

Just as health professionals overestimate our ability to identify noncompliance, we may also overestimate the true impact we have on patients and their medication practice. Zygmunt and colleagues (2002) conducted a systematic literature review of studies testing the impact of psychosocial interventions to improve medication adherence in schizophrenia. Thirteen of thirty-nine (33 percent) studies reported significant intervention effects. In a subgroup analysis of studies that used a random-assignment design and where the study group size was at least ten subjects, six of twenty-three studies (26 percent) showed significant effects of the intervention on medication adherence. They concluded that educational interventions alone typically were not alone in improving medication adherence. To be effective, educational strategies must be accompanied by behavioral and supportive services. Peterson and colleagues (2003) conducted a meta-analysis of randomized controlled trials with at least ten subjects per intervention group. Examples of educational strategies employed in these studies included oral, audiovisual, written, telephoned, mailed means of communicating the message. Behavioral strategies included dosing schedule changes, packaging modification, mail, telephone, and e-mail reminders systems, and others. Overall, the study showed a positive but minimal effect of adherence interventions. Hyperlipidemia was the only medical condition for which a behavioral intervention had a significant effect size. Effect sizes for educational interventions were positive but nonsignificant regardless of disease subgroup cohort. Interventions appeared to improve medication adherence, modestly, with no strategy consistently being superior. Takiya and colleagues (2004) conducted a similar analysis of the interventions to affect medication adherence in hypertension. Results were consistent with the study by Peterson in that the overall effect size for behavioral interventions was small but nonsignificant. Due to the heterogeneity of studies employing educational interventions, effect size was not reported.

The conclusion of these reviews is not that the health professionals and their interventions have little or no effect. Rather, the conclusions serve as a recognition of the fact that patient compliance with medication is a complex issue that we have only begun to understand. Peterson (2003) concludes by stating, "There does not seem to be any one intervention that robustly enhances adherence, perhaps because so many variables affect a patient's decision to take a drug" (p. 65).

Patient and Clinician Perspective

The exchange and interaction between patient and clinician is a complex mix of expectations and assumptions. The same is true of medication as part of the exchange. Clinicians expect that once a medicine is prescribed it will be taken according to directions. The previously cited work by Miller et al. (2002) in which clinicians over-estimated compliance indicates that they assume that patient behavior will coincide with medical advice. However, patients' expectations and assumptions might not be consistent with that of health professional. Conrad (1985) proposes that basic assumptions by patients and clinicians regarding medication compliance are different. Recognizing this difference is essential to understanding patient behavior regarding prescribed therapies. One assumption is that the physiologic parameters clinicians use to assess success and failure of treatment are important to patients. Rather, patients are more interested in how the medical condition or prescribed therapy will affect their ability to function in their numerous roles. Patients are less interested in their thyroid level than in their ability to function at work and home. Unfortunately, these physiologic measures dominate our interaction with patients. We initiate, discontinue, or alter therapy based on these values. From the patient's perspective, they are not rooted in any meaningful way in their everyday lives. The second assumption is that medication compliance is actually important to patients. Compliance is a creation of the health care provider and has little relevance to the patient. Developing strategies to reduce noncompliance is an effort to solve a problem from the clinician's perspective that does not exist the patient's perspective. Patients develop their own medication practice, which may or may not coincide with medical advice. The determinants of this practice are physical, economic, psychological, and social in nature. The degree of compliance may have little to do with medical condition, diagnosis, or the health care provider. The third assumption is that patient values are consistent with clinician values. Clinicians value patients reaching "goal" for the particular medical condition. Patients value the ability to function in their social roles. Gabe and Thorogood (1986) reported that medication was viewed as either enabling or constraining factors for patients as they cope with life. Arluke (1980), in a study of twenty rheumatoid arthritis patients, concluded that medication decisions are based on whether the medication allows patients to reach some desired somatic or behavioral outcome. Conrad (1985) concluded in his study of eighty patients with epilepsy that physical side-effects are not as influential in medication-taking behavior as the social consequence of these side effects. The fourth assumption is that nonadherence represents something wrong. Again, this conceptualization reflects the class of perspective. While noncompliance may be considered wrong from the clinician's perspective, it may be purposeful and understandable from the patient's perspective. Patients develop their medication practice for a variety of reasons. The medicine may be symbolic of external control and the stigma of having a medical condition. Noncompliance may be a way to exert independence and avoid stigma. Patient noncompliance may be an effort to test the limits of their medical condition. There is little reason to take a medicine four times a day if I still get the benefit from taking it once a day. In effect, noncompliance may be a way of verifying that the medical condition is improving or not as severe. Noncompliance may be the observed consequence of patients self-regulating. Conrad argues that what clinicians see as noncompliance, patients see as self-regulation. Patients alter their medication practice depending on the continual feedback they receive and the demand they experience in their lives.

We as health professionals operate from the medical model in our dealings with patients. They, on the other hand, operate from a social model as they make decisions regarding their care. We see them as patients whose decisions should be dictated by this role. They see themselves as people who function in a variety of social roles, and who spend only a brief and at times unrewarding part of that time as patients in a sick role. The degree to which we can escape our perspective, and see the role of medicine in peoples' lives from their perspective, will enhance our ability to affect their medication practice and improve their health outcomes.

MAKE SENSE OF THE VAST
AND CONTRADICTORY LITERATURE

Health professionals today are placed in a quandary. We live in an age where information is abundant and easily accessible, made possible by society's interest in all things related to health, industry's success at creating new products and services, and technology's prowess at making expanded capability affordable. However, the abundance and accessibility of information creates its own problems for health professionals. Davis and colleagues (2004) estimate that over 400,000 articles are added to the biomedical literature each year. Dawes and Sampson (2003) in a review of the literature on information-seeking behavior report that the huge amount of material is one factor in clinicians not seeking information to answer clinical questions. In his aptly named book, *Data Smog,* David Shenk (1997) argues that what we view as a wealth of information is actually an information glut. He offers six laws of data smog, with #6 being, "too many experts spoil the clarity."

And so it is with the field of medication compliance. While much of this book examines appropriately the intricacies of measures and models, the health professional is faced with the question, "what should I do to enhance or sustain medication compliance?" The problem is compounded by the fact that the topic has been explored formally for almost fifty years. For some, this history might be viewed as providing a wealth of information. For others, it might be considered an information glut about which there is little clarity. The field has benefited from periodic reviews, including the work of Sackett and Haynes (1976), Meichenbaum and Turk (1987), and more recently, the meta-analyses of Takiya et al. (2004), Peterson et al. (2003), Vermeire et al. (2005), Schedlbauer, Schroeder, Peters, and Fahey (2005), and Dolder, Lacro, Leckband, and Dilip (2003). Yet, in spite of these reviews, the health care professional may still be faced with competing views as to what works and what does not. Within specific therapeutic categories, the clinical research community responds to these challenges by developing practice guidelines or best practices documents. As medication adherence is an element of practice that crosses both therapeutic and disciplinary lines, developing and implementing best-medication adherence practice guidelines has remained elusive.

In spite of these barriers, health care practitioners develop their own practice with regard to medication compliance. A crucial element in developing an effective medication adherence practice is being a discriminating user of the compliance literature, in the absence of practice guidelines. Nichol and colleagues (1999) examined a random sample of 72 articles from a total of 719 identified via a computer search of the literature. Sixty-four percent of studies were descriptive in nature. The compliance measure or its criteria were stated in only fifty of the seventy-two articles. The authors also developed methodologic scales standardized to range from 0 to 100 to assess the quality of study design issues, disease-related issues, and compliance scores within each study. Median summary scores for the 3 areas were 8.3, 42.9, and 50 respectively. The authors conclude that the average quality of the literature on compliance with medications is poor.

This conclusion is neither isolated nor relegated to a particular period of time. Sackett and Haynes (1976) computed a score reflecting the methodologic rigor of the articles reviewed. While the theoretical range of the scale was 0 to 22, the actual range was 5 to 16, with the mean score being about 10. Bruer (1982) examined the relationship between scale score for articles reviewed by Sackett and Haynes (1976) and citation score as reported by the Science Citation Index and the Social Science Citation Index. He reports a significant but low correlation between scale score and citation ($r = 0.26$), suggesting that the citation score would not be a good indicator of an articles methodological rigor. Of perhaps greater importance to health professionals is the unavoidable conclusion that work of questionable rigor is being published and cited by others, thereby making it difficult to develop an effective, evidenced-based, medication adherence practice. Similar concerns about the suboptimal quality of the compliance literature have been expressed recently by Higgins and Regan (2004), DiMatteo (2004), and Schedlbauer et al. (2005).

Given these limitations, health professionals still must make sense of the information available to them, and must make decisions concerning which elements should be incorporated into their practice. To make sense of the extensive, and sometimes conflicting, information, health care providers must employ some organizing framework to efficiently assimilate the information. Meichenbaum and Turk (1987) have provided a systematic way to understand the factors that may influence medication adherence. They classified all possible factors into one of the following five headings: (1) patient variables, (2) disease variables, (3) treatment variables, (4) organizational-structural variables, and (5) relationship variables (patient and health care provider). Patient variables might include demographic characteristics such as age, gender, or income. Disease variables might examine the influence of comorbidity, or the presence of symptoms, on medication compliance. Treatment variables might include the complexity of therapeutic regimen. Organizational-structural variables might include access to care or burdens of receiving care inherent in the delivery system, for example, hours, co-payments, formularies, and so on. Relationship variables would focus on the quality of relationship between patient and health care provider. This framework recently directed the World Health Organization's examination of adherence with long-term therapies (Sabate, 2003), which concluded that opportunities to improve medication adherence are rooted in patient factors, social and economic factors, condition-related factors, therapy or treatment factors, and health care team and system-related factors. The broader literature provides some support for the contention that specific interventions in each area can be effective in improving medication compliance. For example, patient self-efficacy (patient factor) has been shown to be related to compliance in AIDS (2005), multiple sclerosis (2001), and diabetes (2001). Social support, including nonfamily support (social factor), is related to compliance in depression (2005), AIDS (2004), and in adolescents with chronic disease (2001). The presence of depression as a comorbidity in patients with diabetes (condition-related factor) was associated with lower compliance with both medication and diet regimens (2005). Reducing the frequency of dosing (treatment factor) has been consistently associated with medication compliance (2001). A positive health provider–patient relationship (health care team factor) has been shown to be associated with medication compliance in AIDS (2004) and fibromyalgia (2004).

A more detailed accounting of the methods to impact patient compliance with medication is found in Chapter 7 by Jack Fincham. The purpose of the presentation of the frameworks of Meichenbaum and

Turk (1987) and Sabate's (2003) World Health Report on adherence to long-term therapies is to assist in the assimilation of the vast and inconsistent literature regarding medication compliance. As health providers develop their own strategies to improve the medication compliance within their own patients, this framework will serve to make those efforts more effective and efficient.

COMMITMENT TO THE DEVELOPMENT OF BEST PRACTICES REGARDING MEDICATION ADHERENCE

The concept of best practices assumes that there exists, at the population level, some intervention or combination of interventions that constitute what health providers should do in the face of noncompliance. By definition, implementation of these interventions should benefit the greatest number of patients. The current state of noncompliance argues both for and against the development of best practices or guidelines. The consistently small effect size of the tested interventions, and the conclusion that no one intervention is superior to others, suggests that the development of best practices and guidelines is premature. Furthermore, the health disciplines are far from an adequate understanding of the concept of medication compliance, and are still further from adopting and/or testing competing models from nonmedical disciplines. Lastly, because compliance or noncompliance is a behavior, patient variability in attitude, belief, and behavioral response makes best practices problematic. However, for these very reasons, the time is propitious for such a commitment. The cost and consequence of continued noncompliance has been described previously. Small effect sizes suggest that our current interventions, as conceptualized and implemented, may be inadequate. Our attachment to the medical model has limited our understanding of the meaning of medicine and patients' decisions to follow or not follow recommendation. Expansion of this view is critical. Finally, the inherent variability indicates that best practices serve only as a guide to be tailored to individual patients, requiring greater commitment on the part of health professionals to accommodate patient-specific concerns.

Although the health professional now has a way of organizing the various interventions, he or she must still utilize some filter to separate the studies with greatest impact from those that will not be influential in developing one's own compliance strategies. A reasonable approach to this problem is to utilize the reviews that have employed some methodological criteria in evaluating studies on the effectiveness of interventions to improve medication adherence. Such an approach addresses the concerns listed earlier related to methodological shortcoming of the compliance literature. Studies with stronger designs will minimize the confounding and biases that lead to alternative explanations for results. The expectation of following this process is the emergence of some consistency in the observed results that will further direct and inform the health professional as to what works and what does not. The results can serve as the initial point of departure into best practice dialogue.

Many of the reviews of the literature on medication compliance that employ stringent inclusion criteria classify the interventions as educational, behavioral, or some type of social support, which may include group activity, provider–patient relationship, and so on. Schroeder and colleagues (2004) performed a systematic review of randomized controlled trial to assess the impact of interventions to improve adherence to antihypertensive medications in the ambulatory setting. Only one of six studies using educational strategies alone showed improvement in adherence. Behavioral strategies, specifically, simplification of dosing regimen, showed improvement in adherence in seven of nine studies, with improvement ranging from 8.0 to 19.6 percent. Complex interventions that included combinations of educational, behavioral, and motivational strategies showed improved adherence in eight of eighteen studies. Schedlbauer and colleagues (2005) assessed the effect of interventions directed to improve medication adherence to lipid-lowering drugs by reviewing randomized contrail trials for both primary and secondary prevention of cardiovascular disease in the ambulatory setting. The process of study selection yielded eight studies that satisfied inclusion criteria. Three interventions resulted in significant improvement in adherence: (1) simplification of drug regimen (11 percent improvement in adherence by changing dosing from four times a day to two times a day), (2) information and education (13 percent increase in adherence resulting from pharmacist-provided videotapes, booklets, and newspapers followed by educational newsletters), and (3) patient reminding (24 percent improvement in adherence resulting from weekly phone call reminders). McDonald and colleagues (2002) examined the influence of intervention on medication adherence in unconfounded randomized controlled trials for medical or psychiatric disorders. In three studies that simplified the dosing regimen, significant improvements in medication adherence occurred. Studies that examined the effectiveness of educational interventions reported significant improvements for short-term therapy. Interventions that were successful for long-term therapy were typically complex, including some elements of education, behavioral change, and social support. Dolder et al.'s (2003) review of interventions to improve antipsychotic medication adherence yields similar results, namely, that educational strategies alone were the least successful at improving medication adherence, and that the greatest improvement in adherence is realized through interventions that include educational, behavioral, and affective strategies.

The consistency of the major reviews regarding the effectiveness of interventions to improve medication adherence can serve as the basis of any discussion of best practices. Educational strategies alone have a narrow place in the toolbox to improve medication adherence, namely, for short-term medical conditions. For longer-term conditions and treatments, education is necessary but not sufficient for improved adherence. The most effective strategies include educational, behavioral, and affective/social support components. The behavioral strategy that appears to be the most consistent element of a successful strategy to improve adherence is reducing regimen complexity. The multifaceted nature of the interventions strongly suggests the need for interdisciplinary approaches.

RECENT TRENDS IN COMPLIANCE RESEARCH

The traditional view of interdisciplinary interventions is that each health professional functions within his or her expected roles to contribute to a coordinated team effort. Recently published studies in the area of medication compliance point to an expansion of the traditional roles that health professional play. The reported consistency in improving medication adherence suggests a dynamic between health professional and patient that should be explored further.

The effectiveness of pharmacists in improving medication compliance in primary care settings has been evaluated in several studies. Bouvy and colleagues (2003) conducted a randomized controlled study in which patients were assigned to pharmacist-led interventions on medication compliance in patients with heart failure, and usual care. Intervention consisted of a structured interview between pharmacist and patient that included discussion about the medication, reasons for noncompliance, and difficulties of incorporating medication use into the patient's daily life. Monthly follow-up contact was initiated by the pharmacist and repeated over a period of six months. The risk of a one-day or two-day gap in therapy due to noncompliance was significantly less in the intervention group. Sookaneknun and colleagues (2004) assessed the effectiveness of pharmacist involvement in two primary care clinics for patient with hypertension. Subjects were randomized to pharmacist involvement groups or to traditional service. The intervention consisted of a thirty- to fifty-minute consultation that addressed disease, treatment, adherence, and lifestyle issues related to hypertension. Patients received written educational leaflets at the initial consultation, and revisited the pharmacist monthly. Reductions in both systolic and diastolic pressures were significantly greater in the intervention group. A significantly greater proportion of patients with elevated blood pressure in the intervention group had controlled systolic and diastolic pressures post intervention than in the control group. Similar results are reported in studies examining pharmacist primary care interventions in dyslipidemia (Ali, Lauren, Lariviere, Tremblay, & Cloutier, 2003), obesity (Malone & Alger-Mayer, 2003), and diabetes (Nowak, Singh, Clarke, Campbell, & Jaber, 2002). One non-confirming study by Odegard and colleagues (2005) reported that a pharmacist intervention that included the development of a diabetes care plan and weekly pharmacist–patient communication showed no benefit in medication compliance over the control group.

The role of nurses is expanding beyond the more traditional institutional settings. Nurses are directing and managing disease-management programs for high-risk patients with a variety of chronic conditions.

Patients remain in their home and community, but their care is managed by nurses who either visit or contact them via telephone. Rudd and colleagues (2004) randomized patients needing therapy for hypertension to usual medical care or usual medical care plus nurse care management intervention. An initial counseling session with the nurse care manager included educational and behavioral interventions such as information on the correct use of an automated blood pressure device, suggestions to enhance medication adherence, and recognition of possible side effects. Follow-up phone contacts occurred at one week, one, two, and four months. Both systolic and diastolic readings were significantly lower in the nurse care manager group than usual medical care group. In addition, medication adherence was significantly better in the nurse care manager group (80.5 percent versus 69.2 percent) than in the usual medical care group. Bosworth and colleagues (2005) examined the effect of nurse-administered patient-tailored telephone calls to patients with hypertension. The intervention included modules on a variety of topics, for example, hypertension knowledge, medication refills, health behaviors, social support, patient–provider communication, and others. Modules were provided via telephone communication between patient and nurse every other month, or monthly, if a problem arose. Preliminary results of this two-year study show that 46 percent of the patients randomized to nurse intervention who were nonadherent at baseline were adherent at six months. Thirty-four percent of patients in the usual care group who were nonadherent at baseline were adherent at six months (p = 0.08).

The importance of these nontraditional roles for pharmacists and nurses reported earlier is not the effectiveness of the intervention. Rather, the nurse and pharmacists are functioning in a novel capacity for the patient in a way that expands the patient–provider relationship. While much has been written about the relationship, its relationship to medication adherence has not been fully explored. Most adherence interventions include a health provider. The effectiveness of face-to-face counseling, recommendations to alter existing therapy, referral to more intensive care, all involve the participation of the health professional. Yet, given the current system where providers function in traditional roles, the effectiveness of adherence interventions is underwhelming. This trend of health professionals of expanding the nature of their contact with patients may be cause to reconsider the role of the patient–provider relationship in adherence.

SUMMARY

This chapter was motivated by a belief that health providers have a professional responsibility to assist patients to achieve positive health outcomes. For many people, these outcomes are made possible through adherence with prescribed therapy. The second motivation was to discuss the role of the health professional in medication compliance, without reiterating the information presented in other chapters. The goal was to raise specific questions or concerns for the reader to consider within the context of health professionals' contribution to medication adherence. The first issue was for physicians, nurses, and pharmacists to recognize our own limitations and bias. We must know that we are not adept at identifying noncompliant patients, we must acknowledge the limits of our influence, and we must recognize the discordance between our perspective and the patient's perspective. Second, we must utilize some organizing framework to effectively and efficiently use the growing literature that supports health care practice. And third, we should consider whether this particular time in the development of our knowledge and limitations regarding medication compliance is appropriate to consider best practices and clinical guidelines for a medication compliance practice. Finally, the reader is asked to consider the patient–provider relationship, especially in light of emerging practice roles.

REFERENCES

Ali, F., Lauren, M. Y., Lariviere, C., Tremblay, D., & Cloutier, D. (2003). The effect of pharmacist intervention and patient education on lipid-lowering medication compliance and plasma cholesterol levels. *Can J Clin Pharm, 10*(3):101-106.

Arluke, A. (1980). Judging drugs: Patients' conceptions of therapeutic efficacy in the treatment of arthritis. *Human Org, 39*(1): 84-88.

Bosworth, H. B., Olsen, M. K., Gentry, P., Orr, M., Dudley, T., McCant, F., & Oddone, E. Z. (2005). Nurse administered telephone intervention for blood pressure control: A patient-tailored multi-factorial intervention. *PatEduc Couns, 57*(1): 5-14.

Bouvy, M. L., Heerdink, E. R., Urquhart, J., Grobbee, D., Hoe, A. W., & Leufkens, H. G. M. (2003). Effect of a pharmacist-led intervention on diuretic compliance in heart failure patients: A randomized controlled study. *J Card Fail, 9:* 404-411.

Bruer, J. T. (1982). Methodolgical rigor and citation frequency in patient compliance literature. *Am J Publ Health, 72:* 1119-1123.

Conrad, P. (1985). The meaning of medicine: Another look at compliance. *Soc Sci Med, 20*(1): 29-37.

Davis, D. A., Ciurea, I., Flanagan, T. M., & Perrier, L. (2004). Solving the information overload problem: A letter from Canada. *Med J Aust, 180*(6): S68-S71.

Dawes, M. & Sampson, U. (2003). Knowledge management in clinical practice: A systematic review of information seeking behavior in physicians. *International J Med Inf, 71:* 9-15.

DiMatteo, M. R. (2004). Variation in patients' adherence to medical recommendations: A quantitative review of 50 years of research. *Med Care, 42:* 200-209.

Dolder, C. R., Lacro, J. P., Leckband, S., & Dilip, J. (2003). Interventions to improve antipsychotic medication adherence: Review of recent literature. *J Clin Psychopharm, 23*(4): 389-399.

Gabe, J. & Thorogood, N. (1986). Prescribed drug use and the management of everyday life: The experiences of black and white working-class women. *Soc Rev, 34:* 737-772.

Higgins, N. & Regan, C. (2004). A systematic review of the effectiveness of interventions to help older people adhere to medication regimens. *Age Ageing, 33:* 224-229.

McDonald, H. P., Garg, A. X., & Haynes, R. B. (2002). Interventions to enhance patient adherence to medication prescriptions. *JAMA, 288:* 2868-2879.

Malone, M. & Alger-Mayer, S. A. (2003). Pharmacist intervention enhances adherence to Orlistat therapy. *Ann Pharmacother, 37:* 1598-1602.

Meichenbaum, D. & Turk, D. C. (1987). *Facilitating treatment adherence* (pp. 203-217). New York: Plenum Press.

Miller, L. G., Honghu, L., Hays, R., Golin, C., Beck, C. K., Asch, S. M., Ma, Y., Kaplan, A., & Wenger, N. (2002). How well do clinicians estimate patients' adherence to combination antiretroviral therapy? *J Gen Int Med, 17:* 1-11.

Nichol, M. B., Venturini, F., & Sung, J. C. Y. (1999). A critical evaluation of the methodology of the literature on medication compliance. *Ann Pharmacother, 33:* 531-540.

Nowak, S. N., Singh, R., Clarke, A., Campbell, E., & Jaber, L. A. (2002). Metabolic control and adherence to American Diabetes Association Practice Guidelines in a pharmacist-managed diabetes clinic. *Diab Care, 25:* 1479.

Odegard, P. S., Goo, A., Williams, K. L., & Gray, S. L. (2005). Caring for poorly controlled diabetes mellitus: A randomized pharmacist intervention. *Ann Pharmacother, 39:* 433-440.

Peterson, A. M., Takiya, L., & Finley, R. (2003). Meta-analysis of trials of interventions to improve medication adherence. *Am J Health Sys Pharm, 60:* 657-665.

Rudd, P., Miller, N. H., Kaufman, J., Kraemer, H. C., Bandura, A., Greenwald, G., & Debusk, R. F. (2004). Nurse management for hypertension. *American Journal of Hypertension, 17:* 921-927.

Sabate, E. (2003). Adherence to long-term therapies: Evidence for action. Geneva: World Health Organization.

Sackett, D. L. & Haynes, R. B. (1976). *Compliance with therapeutic regimens* (pp. 3-23). Baltimore: The Johns Hopkins Press.

Schedlbauer, A., Schroeder, K., Peters, T. J., & Fahey, T. (2005). Interventions to improve adherence to lipid lowering medication. *The Cochrane Database of Systematic Reviews, 3.* DOI : 10.1002/14651858.CD004371.pub2.

Schroeder, K., Fahey, T., & Ebrahim, S. (2004). How can we improve adherence to blood pressure-lowering medication in ambulatory care? *Arch Int Med, 164:* 722-732.

Shenk, D. (1997). *Data smog: Surviving the information glut* (pp. 23-37). New York: HarperCollins.

Sookaneknun, P., Richards, R. M. E., Sanguansermsri, J., & Teeasut C. (2004). Pharmacist involvement in primary care improves hypertensive patient clinical outcomes. *Ann Pharmacother, 38:* 2023-2028.

Takiya, L., Peterson, A. M., & Finley, R. S. (2004). Meta-analysis of interventions for medication adherence to antihypertensives. *Ann Pharmacother, 38:* 1617-1624.

Vermeire, E., Wens, J., Van Royen, P., Biot, Y., Hearnshaw, H., & Lindenmeyer, A. (2005). Interventions for improving adherence to treatment recommendations in people with type 2 diabetes mellitus. *The Cochrane Database of Systematic Reviews, 3.* DOI : 10.1002/14651858.CD003638.pub2.

Zygmunt, A., Olfson, M., Boyer, C., & Mechanic, D. (2002). Interventions to improve medication adherence in schizophrenia. *Am J Psychiat, 159:* 1653-1664.

Chapter 11

Disease State Management in Older Persons with Hyperlipidemia

Louis Roller
Jenny Gowan

This chapter attempts to outline the complexity in treating older persons with risk factors for cardiovascular and/or cerebrovascular disease, with particular emphasis on hyperlipidemia. This is illustrated by means of a case study highlighting the importance of patient compliance with lipid-lowering therapies and dietary guidelines.

Most Americans can expect to live relatively long and healthy lives. An American boy born between 2000 and 2001 can expect to live on average 75.0 years, and a girl born in the same period can expect to live 80.3 years (CDC, 2005), which compares well with most other developed countries. The Japanese have the longest life expectancy of 77.3 years for men and 84.1 years for women. To put this in context, compare the life expectancies of Indians (the subcontinent) of 62.4 years for men and 63.3 years for women (Yahoo, 2005).

In 2000, people sixty-five years onward formed about 12.4 percent of the U.S. population, which is approximately 35 million people which in turn is nearly twice the total population of Australia (U.S. Census Bureau, 2003), but consume a disproportionate number of medications. It has been estimated that older persons will constitute 20.7 percent (or 87 million) by the year 2050 (U.S. Census Bureau, 2004). Older persons have some special problems with the use of medications. They are at particular risk if they have multiple medical

Patient Compliance with Medications: Issues and Opportunities
© 2007 by The Haworth Press, Inc. All rights reserved.
doi:10.1300/5365_11

problems and are taking multiple medications. It is not surprising, therefore, that older people experience adverse drug reactions more often than younger people (Barraclough, 2002; Lasarou, Pomeranz, & Corey, 1998; Roughead, 1999) and struggle with patient compliance.

Apart from the changes in drug response caused by pharmacokinetic alterations, older persons may differ from younger people in their sensitivity to drugs. They are often more sensitive to the effects of drugs (Beers, 2000; Koda-Kimble et al., 2005). Older people may have an impaired *homeostatic* mechanism to protect against orthostatic hypotension. Slipping, tripping, poor balance, and weak legs contribute to almost 80 percent of falls with dizziness and fainting accounting for another 6 percent. Falls are commonly caused by gait and balance disorders, weakness, environmental hazards, confusion, arthritis, visual impairment, and postural hypotension.

Adverse effects of many drugs may increase an individual's risk of falls. Combinations of any of these agents will further increase risk plus environmental factors. Table 11.1 summarizes adverse effects of some groups of drugs that may increase risk of falls.

Hypnotics, anxiolytics, and other CNS depressant drugs may cause confusion, incontinence, and unsteady gait, which may cause falls and fractures. Barbiturates and benzodiazepine hypnotics have been overused in the past, especially in hostels and nursing homes. The use of nondrug sleep hygiene methods is preferable. Long-acting benzodiazepines, for example, diazepam, nitrazepam, should be avoided in older persons as they may continue to exert the adverse effects and, therefore, lead to significant morbidity in older patients.

Confusion may be caused by many commonly used drugs, including the H_2-antagonists, particularly in older patients with diminished renal function (Beers, 2000; Koda-Kimble et al., 2005).

Nonsteroidal antiinflammatory drugs (NSAIDS) including COX-2 inhibitors should be used with great care in older patients, since there is an increased risk of peptic ulceration and adverse effects on renal and cardiac function. In addition, these drugs may cause dizziness, which may lead to falls and fractures (Johnsen et al., 2005).

Use of Cox-2 inhibitors (celecoxib and rofecoxib, etc.) was thought to be of some value in older persons who could not tolerate traditional NSAIDs due to gastrointestinal adverse effects. The Cox-2 inhibitors may elicit a similar range of adverse reactions to the traditional

TABLE 11.1. Adverse effects of drugs that may increase risk of falls.

Adverse effect	Drug class
Blurred vision	Anticholinergics
	Eye ointments
Cerebellar dysfunction	Alcohol
	Anticonvulsants
Drowsiness or sedation	Alcohol
	Antidepressants especially tricyclics
	Anticonvulsants
	Antihistamines—first generation
	Antipsychotics
	Anxiolytics and hypnotics (e.g. benzodiazepines)
	Major tranquillizers
	Opioid analgesics
Parkinsonism	Antiemetics
	Major tranquillizers
	Vestibular suppressants
Postural hypotension	Antihypertensives, especially methyldopa, alpha blockers (e.g. prazosin, doxazosin, terazosin, tamsulosin, and alfuzosin)
	Antidepressants especially tricylic antidepressants
	Diuretics, e.g., furosemide
	Drugs for Parkinson's disease
	NSAIDs

Source: Adapted from Hill, K., & Schwarz J. (2001). The impact of falls on older people: How to assess the risks and implement prevention strategies. In Clunig, T. (Ed.), *Ageing at Home* (pp. 131-155). Sansom, L. N. (2004). *Australian Pharmaceutical Formulary* (19th ed). Canberra: Pharmaceutical Society of Australia, Canberra.

NSAIDs and also increase the risk of cardiovascular disease (Therapeutic Guidelines, 2002). The drug of choice in the treatment of osteoarthritis in older persons is acetaminophen 650 to 1000 mg equivalent four times a day (Beers, 2000; Semal, Beixer, & Higby 2001; USP-DI, 2005).

Drugs with anticholinergic effects (e.g., tricyclic antidepressants and some antiparkinsonian drugs, as well as some nonprescription medications), may cause the well-known range of anticholinergic side effects including constipation, blurred vision, confusion, and urinary retention (of special concern in older male patients who may have prostate problems).

Older people are very sensitive to the hypoglycemic effects of glibenclamide (and other long-acting hypoglycemics), due in part to pharmacokinetic alterations. This drug may lead to a potentially dangerous, pronounced, and prolonged lowering of blood sugar concentration in older people (Beers, 2000, 1995; Semal, Beixer, & Higby 2001; USP-DI, 2005)

Theophylline has a low therapeutic index and has been shown to cause cardiac arrhythmias in people (especially older ones) even within the therapeutic range. If the drug must be used, plasma theophylline concentrations should be monitored at regular intervals and the dosage individualized (Beers, 2000; USP-DI, 2005).

The antibiotic combination, trimethoprim/sulfamethoxazole, has been associated with an increased risk of serious adverse reactions in older people, including bone marrow depression and serious skin reactions (Beers, 2000; USP-DI, 2005) and unless there are no other alternatives, it should not be used in older persons.

A number of physiologic changes occur with aging and these may modify the absorption (marginal), distribution, hepatic metabolism, and renal excretion of drugs. Many drugs are cleared more slowly in the older person (Beers, 2000; USP-DI, 2005). In particular, the age-related decline in kidney function may lead to a decrease in the renal clearance of drugs and their metabolites. This is important for those drugs that are predominantly renally cleared (e.g., digoxin, fluoroquinolone antimicrobials, fluconazole, ACE inhibitors, and others) or that have a renally cleared active metabolite (e.g., allopurinol). Special care is required in using these drugs, particularly if the drugs have a narrow therapeutic range (Beers, 2000; Semal, Beixer, & Higby, 2001).

In general, *older patients require smaller drug doses.* It must be recognized, however, that physiologic variability increases with age and, therefore, the dosage regimens must be individualized (Lazarou, Pomeranz, & Corey, 1998; Roughead, 1999). In order to best impact noncompliance, this is imperative.

Of particular concern is the "triple whammy effect." Angiotensin Converting Enzyme Inhibitors (ACEI) or Angiotensin II receptor antagonists (AIIRA), NSAIDs and diuretics, individually or in combination, are implicated in over 50 percent of cases of iatrogenic acute renal failure. Wherever possible, NSAIDs should be avoided in patients with chronic renal failure, congestive heart failure, and hypertension, particularly if these patients are also taking ACE inhibitors and/or diuretics. Monitoring of renal function should follow any change in dose of ACE inhibitor or diuretic (Thomas, 2000).

Many older people may be suffering from multiple disease states. This has a number of potential consequences:

- The diseases may effect disposition and drug response.
- Although principles of rational drug therapy discourage polypharmacy, in some cases the addition of another medication or medications may be necessary to prevent an adverse effect, for example, folic acid supplementation in patients taking phenytoin; use of combined antihypertensive agents; potassium supplementation with furosemide, or the use of multi-antimicrobial therapy in the treatment of certain infectious diseases such as tuberculosis and HIV, etc. Problems with noncompliance may, however, be compounded because of increased medication regimen complexity.
- Many drugs produce adverse effects that do not require treatment with other drugs, but require either a dose reduction, drug cessation, and/or drug substitution.
- Many studies have shown that when more drugs are added to the medication program, adherence is adversely affected. This is further complicated by the proliferation of generic brands for which patients may not recognize duplicative therapies.
- The potential for drug interactions and adverse drug reactions increases substantially as the number of drugs taken increases (Lazarou, Pomeranz, & Corey, 1998; Roughead, 1999).

There are many factors that may compromise the ability of older people to use their medicines as intended. Either over- or under-compliance or adherence with the use of drugs may lead to a suboptimal clinical outcome and increase the risk of adverse drug reactions (Horowitz & Horowitz, 1993).

The complexity of the therapeutic regimen is an obvious factor that affects adherence. This is an important, but not the only, reason to avoid complex regimens involving multiple drugs. Older people may have cognitive impairment, memory loss, and confusion (possibly drug-induced), which may seriously affect their ability to understand the prescribers' and pharmacists' counseling instructions about the appropriate use of medicines.

Many older persons find it difficult, if not impossible, to open some medicine containers or to operate certain devices (e.g., metered-dose aerosol inhalers) as a result of muscle weakness (especially in people suffering from arthritis) and poor coordination (Parkinson's disease).

Medication duplication (different and duplicative brands) is a particular risk when patients return to their community after a stay in a hospital or aged care home.

An additional complication may arise for those older people who live alone and, therefore, do not have immediate assistance with their medication (Roller & Gowan, 2000). The use of a dose administration device (compliance packaging, reminders, etc.) may allow these people to remain in their own homes. The care taken to ensure the best therapeutic outcome for patients applies to every aspect of pharmaceutical practice, including, hostels, nursing homes, hospitals and community pharmacies.

Medication management reviews are now considered a vital part of the role of the pharmacist in conjunction with the patient and the prescriber and include the following:

- Need for each current medicine
- Appropriate duration of therapy
- Clinically relevant drug interactions
- Side effects and adverse drug reactions
- Drug-disease interactions (contra-indications)
- Suitability of doses and dosage intervals
- Complexity of the medication program
- Adequacy of instructions
- Patient compliance and the need for compliance aids
- Duplication of different brands of the same drug or different drugs from the same pharmacologic/therapeutic class (DiPiro et al., 1999; Hanlon, Shimp, & Semla, 2000; Koda-Kimble et al., 2005; O Mahony & Martin, 1999)

In Australia, government funding has allowed the development of this role with over 60,000 reviews being conducted in the first 3 years of the program. Figures are now rapidly increasing as the general practitioners realize the benefits of pharmacists working in a team approach to visit the home and to identify what medicines people are actually taking, the difficulties experienced, and to help in risk reduction.

Cardiovascular disease (CVD) accounts for an excess of 930,000 deaths and $350 billion in direct medical costs and lost productivity in the United States each year. CVD accounts for in excess of 930,000 deaths and $350 billion in direct medical costs and lost productivity each year (AHA, 2006).

Numerous clinical trials and meta-analyses have concluded that antihypertensive and lipid-lowering medications substantially reduce the risk of coronary heart disease (CHD), stroke, and death in patients with CVD risk factors (ALLHAT, 2002; Law, Wald, Morris, & Jordan, 2003; Law, Wald, & Rudnicka, 2003; Neal, MacMahon, & Chapman, 2000; Pignone, Phillips, & Mulrow, 2000; Ross et al., 1999; Sever et al., 2003) with long-term therapy yielding the greatest benefit.

The concept of risk factors constitutes a major advance for developing strategies for preventing CHD. The Framingham Heart Study played a vital role in defining the contribution of risk factors to CHD occurrence in the general population of the United States. The major risk factors studied extensively in the study include the following:

- Cigarette smoking
- Hypertension
- High serum cholesterol and various cholesterol fractions
- Low levels of high-density lipoprotein (HDL) cholesterol
- Diabetes mellitus
- Age (men > fifty-five years, women > sixty-five years)
- Noncompliance

Factors other than those listed as *major* risk factors increase the likelihood of developing CHD. Among these, those that have been studied at Framingham or elsewhere are as follows:

- Obesity
- Physical inactivity or sedentary lifestyle
- Family history of premature CHD
- Hypertriglyceridemia
- Small low-density lipoprotein (LDL) particles
- Increased lipoprotein (a) (Lp[a])
- Increased serum homocysteine
- Abnormalities in several coagulation factors. Despite the potential importance of these other factors, they are not included in

the Framingham risk charts for both theoretical and practical reasons (ALLHAT, 2002; Law, Wald, & Rudnicka, 2003; Law et al., 2003; Neal, MacMahon, & Chapman, 2000; Pignone, Phillips, & Mulrow, 2000; Ross et al., 1999; Sever et al., 2003).

Hyperlipidemia or dyslipidemia is a major risk factor for the pathological processes that are responsible for cardiovascular disease. High plasma concentrations of low LDL lead to their retention in the arterial subendothelial space where they may cause a self-perpetuating inflammatory process, which leads to the formation of atherosclerotic plaque (Beers, 2000; Koda-Kimble et al., 2005; Sever et al., 2003). HDL in removing excess cholesterol from peripheral tissues may oppose this process. Unless the excessive levels of LDL and other risk factors are controlled, the plaque will progress to the point where it becomes unstable and ruptures (Beers, 2000; Koda-Kimble et al., 2005). This could precipitate a superimposed thrombosis, which is likely to cause major clinical events such as the acute coronary syndrome. Recommended levels depend on the overall risk for the individual, but LDL cholesterol (LDL-C) levels greater than 200 mg/dL (5.2 mmol/L) are excessive, even in subjects without other risk factors (Sever et al., 2003).

Management principles of hyperlipidemia include provision of *healthy diet and lifestyle* advice, reduction of consumption of saturated and transunsaturated fats (should be less than 10 percent of energy), reduction of dietary cholesterol (should be less than 300 mg/day) and instigation of exercise (it has been shown that walking reduces LDL-C and TC/HDL-C in adults independent of changes in body composition), and caloric restriction (especially in terms of fat and alcohol) and the inclusion of appropriate amounts of plant sterol supplemented foods, such as particular margarines (may be of substantial benefit, further lowering LDL-C by about 10 percent) (Kelley, Kelley, & Tran, 2004; O'Neill et al., 2004).

Drug-induced dyslipidemia may be exacerbated by drugs such as thiazide diuretics, beta-blockers (non-ISA-intrinsic sympathetic activity), estrogens, progestogens, corticosteroids, anabolic steroids, cyclosporine, isotretinoin), and others (Koda-Kimble et al., 2005).

About half of all American adults, regardless of ethnicity, have total cholesterol levels over 200 mg/dL. Over 25 percent have been told by doctors that they have unhealthy levels. The major risk factor for these high rates may be the Western lifestyle. The typical high-fat low-fiber American diet coupled with sedentary habits is largely responsible for this unfortunate trend. Heart disease is the major cause of death in men. On average, men develop coronary artery disease ten to fifteen years earlier than women do and their risk for dying of heart disease at younger ages than women is higher (AHA, 2006a,b; CDC, 2005; O'Mahoney & Martin, 1999).

Coronary artery disease is still the number one cause of death of women as well. Women between the ages of twenty and thirty-four and after menopause, around age fifty-five, have higher cholesterol levels than do men. Some evidence suggests that HDL levels might have more significance in women than in men. In one study, at total cholesterol levels above 200 mg/dL, women with HDL levels below 50 mg/dL had a higher death rate than those with levels above 50 mg/dL, regardless of their LDL cholesterol levels. Women also appear to be more susceptible to the high-triglyceride low-HDL syndrome, which may be a particular risk factor for heart disease.

Obesity is at epidemic levels in all age groups in the United States. The effect of obesity on cholesterol levels is complex. Although obesity does not appear to be strongly associated with overall cholesterol levels, among obese individuals triglyceride levels are usually high while HDL levels tend to be low, both risk factors for heart disease. Obesity, in any case, has other effects (hypertension, increase in inflammation) that pose major risks to the heart.

The effects of high cholesterol, and its treatment, in people over seventy and have been controversial issues. A number of studies report that in older adults, high cholesterol levels pose a significant risk for death from coronary artery disease, while some others have suggested that lowering cholesterol levels in older persons may increase the risk for stroke or heart attack. For example, a 2001 study reported that statin therapy reduces mortality rates in people over sixty-five with heart disease. According to 2000 data, men over seventy years old with levels under 160 mg/dL or over 240 mg/dL were at significant risk for serious heart events. Some experts, then, now suggest that the ideal cholesterol range for older adults may be between 200 and 219 mg/dL (AHA, 2006a,b; O'Mahoney & Martin, 1999; Pignone et al., 2000). ·

LIPID-LOWERING AGENTS

HMG-CoA reductase inhibitors or statins (atorvastatin, fluvastatin, lovastatin, pravastatin, rosuvastatin, and simvastatin) inhibit cholesterol synthesis, thereby increasing LDL receptor-mediated uptake (see Table 11.2). They also reduce triglyceride levels and increase HDL-C levels modestly. Statins are very well tolerated, but may rarely cause myositis, especially if given with drugs that share their particular cytochrome P450 metabolic (CYP3A4) pathway (Beers, 2000; Koda-Kimble et al., 2005; Tatro, 2004; USP-DI, 2005). Care is required in patients receiving fibrates, cyclosporine, imidazole antifungal agents (ketoconazole, itraconazole, fluconazole, voriconazole), macrolide antibiotics (erythromycin, clarithromycin), and possibly niacin or nicotinic acid. This problem is less likely to occur with pravastatin as it is not metabolized through the CYP3A4 isoenzyme pathway (Tatro, 2004).

Statins may also cause elevation of hepatocellular liver function tests (less than 2 percent of patients). Over the last decade or so, there have been several well-designed studies of interventions that principally lower LDL-C. All of these studies, involving no fewer than 2,000 people (often much larger cohorts), over a minimum time of 4 years have consistently shown reductions of about 30 percent in the relative risk of heart attack or death from cardiovascular or cerebrovascular events (Beers, 2000; Koda-Kimble et al., 2005; USP-DI, 2005).

Bile acid sequestering resins (cholestyramine, colestipol) potentiate the action of statins. They prevent bile acid resorption. This re-

TABLE 11.2. Average effects of selected drugs on lipoprotein cholesterol and cholesterol.

Group	LDL	HDL	Triglycerides
Resins	−15-30%	±3%	+3-10%
Ezetimibe	−18-22%	+0-2%	−0.5%
Niacin	−15-30%	+20-35%	−30-60%
Statins	−25-60%	+5-15%	−10-45%
Fibrates	±10-25%	+10-30%	−30-60%

Sources: Adapted from Beers, M. H. et al. (2000). *The Merck manual of geriatrics* (3rd ed). White House Station, NJ: Merck Research laboratories. Koda-Kimble, M. A., Young, L. Y., & Kradjan, W. A. (2005). *Applied therapeutics: The clinical use of drugs* (8th ed). Philadelphia: Lippincott Williams & Wilkins. *USP DI-Volume I: Drug information for the health care professional* (25th ed). Greenwood Village, CO: Thomson MICROMEDEX.

sults in hepatic depletion of precursor cholesterol, which leads to increased LDL uptake by hepatic LDL receptors. Resins are not systemically absorbed, so their side effects and drug interactions are limited to the gastrointestinal tract, for example, bloating, dyspepsia, and constipation. Although the safety and efficacy of monotherapy with resins are well established, they are mainly reserved for combination therapy with statins in cases of resistant hypercholesterolemia and also, due to adverse effects, have a low patient acceptance (Beers, 2000; Koda-Kimble et al., 2005; USP-DI, 2005).

Niacin (also known as nicotinic acid) reduces fatty acid release from peripheral adipose tissue, thereby reducing the synthesis of very low-density lipoproteins (VLDL). It reduces cholesterol, triglyceride, and lipoprotein, and increases HDL-C. It is difficult to tolerate due to flushing (which may be reduced by gradual dosage escalation and prior use of aspirin) and may cause hyperuricemia, hyperglycaemia, gastritis and, at high doses, hepatitis (Beers, 2000; Koda-Kimble et al., 2005; USP-DI, 2005).

Ezetimibe reduces absorption of dietary and biliary cholesterol and other sterols by inhibiting its transport across the intestinal wall. This leads to an increased demand for cholesterol, an increase in LDL uptake, and its removal from the plasma (Beers, 2000; Koda-Kimble et al., 2005; USP-DI, 2005).

Fibrates (fenofibrate, gemfibrozil) stimulate the alpha peroxisome proliferator activated receptor system that coordinates the expression of genes that catabolize fatty acids and triglycerides. As a result, they reduce VLDL and triglyceride whilst they increase HDL-C. They may increase LDL particle size and, in the process, LDL-C levels sometimes increase rather than decrease. Side effects of fibrates are infrequent but include cholelithiasis, myositis, and increased liver function tests (LFTs). They potentiate coumarin anticoagulants. Clinical trials show angiographic and outcome benefits, but these may be underestimates because they have yet to be tested in a suitable group of patients with mild-to-moderate hypertriglyceridemia (Beers, 2000; Koda-Kimble et al., 2005; USP-DI, 2005). Fenofibrate is given in daily doses of 67 to 160 mg. Three of the 67 mg capsules (201 mg) are considered to be bioequivalent to one of the 160 mg tablets (USP-DI, 2005).

The omega-3 fatty acid component of fish oil preparations reduces hepatic triglyceride synthesis. A dose of 2 to 5 g of the omega-3-fatty acid (6 to 15 g of fish oil) lowers triglyceride. Fish oils also alter thromboxane and prostacyclin metabolism. Omega-3 fatty acids are credited with substantial protection against CHD death. A recent study has found that among individuals aged seventy to ninety years, adherence to a Mediterranean diet (high in omega-3-fatty acids) and healthy lifestyle is associated with a more than 50 percent lower rate of all-causes and cause-specific mortality (Knoops et al., 2004). Table 11.2 lists common lipid-lowering drugs and approximate efficacies in decreasing low-density cholesterol, triglycerides, and in increasing high-density cholesterol.

The "statins" are the mainstay of the treatment for hyperlipidemia. There is, however, a significant correlation between risk factors and the development of rhabdomyolysis (Tatro, 2004). Risk factors include the following:

- Concomitant CYP3A4 inhibitors (such as cyclosporine, diltiazem, verapamil, macrolide antibiotics, imidazole antifungals, protease inhibitors, grapefruit juice [Tatro, 2004])
- Concomittant gemfibrozil/fenofibrate
- Disease states (diabetes, hypothyroidism, renal and hepatic disease)
- Age (>seventy years) and high statin dose (>40 mg/day)

Rhabdomyolysis is the breakdown of muscle fibers resulting in the release of muscle fiber contents into the circulation, causing possible renal damage and/or failure. Symptoms include abnormal urine color (dark, red, or cola-colored), muscle tenderness, weakness of the affected muscle(s), generalized weakness, muscle stiffness, or aching (myalgia). Additional symptoms that may be associated with this disease include weight gain (unintentional), seizures, joint pain, and fatigue (Beers, 2000).

ADHERENCE TO LIPID-LOWERING THERAPY

Studies have shown that, even if patients are managed appropriately, many will discontinue their own treatment. Australian studies in 1994 and again in 1999 demonstrated extremely high levels of medication discontinuance (35 to 60 percent within three to twelve months). The significant predictors of discontinuation were older age and not living in a capital city (Simons, Levis, & Simons, 1996; Simons, Simons, McManus, & Dudley, 2000). Large studies carried out in the United States, Scandinavia, and France obtained similar results. Adherence with concomitant antihypertensive and lipid-lowering therapy is poor, with only one in three patients adherent with both antihypertensive and hypolipidemic medications at six months. Physicians may be able to significantly improve adherence by initiating antihypertensive and antihyperlipidemic concomitantly and by reducing the number of medications being taken (Kiortsis, Giral, Bruckert, & Turpin, 2000). Currently, there are many fixed-dose combination products containing such medications as a statin plus ezetimibe, a statin plus low-dose aspirin, a statin plus an antihypertensive agent (not available in the United States). These combinations are designed to reduce costs to the consumer and, equally importantly, to improve adherence.

An interesting article of a meta-analysis of hundreds of studies was used to determine the combination of drugs for use in a single daily tablet to achieve a large effect in preventing cardiovascular disease with minimal adverse effects. The strategy was to simultaneously reduce four cardiovascular risk factors (LDL-cholesterol, BP, serum homocysteine, and platelet function) regardless of pretreatment levels.

It was found that the formulation that met the objectives was as follows: a statin (atorvastatin 10 mg daily or simvastatin, 40 mg); three blood pressure lowering drugs (e.g., a thiazide, a beta-blocker, and an ACEI), each at half standard dose; folic acid (0.8 mg); and aspirin (75 mg).

It was estimated that the combination (Polypill) would reduce ischaemic heart disease (IHD) events by 88 percent and stroke by 80 percent. One-third of people taking this medication from age fifty-five would benefit, gaining on average about eleven years of life free from an IHD event or stroke (Wald & Law, 2003).

SCENARIO

Mr. David Crockett, a regular and frequent client in your pharmacy, comes in today and hands you a prescription for meloxicam 15 mg, one daily and indicates that he would also like something for his constipation. He knows that you have his full medication and medical history and he sees you as a trusted professional. He also gives you his latest laboratory results (see Table 11.3) as is his habit.

He complains of muscle aches and pains for which the regular physician had suggested increasing the dose of meloxicam to 15 mg. He tells you that the chest discomfort (he refuses to call it pain) has moderated somewhat since going on the diltiazem, but this new medicine does tend to make him constipated. Also, he feels very lethargic. However, his general practitioner (GP) is well pleased with the way his lipids are going, and is not concerned about the increases in liver enzymes. Mr. Crockett also indicates that his urine has developed a brownish color over the last few weeks.

Background

Mr. Crockett has had four coronary arterial grafts eight years ago, a coronary stent put in some four years ago, and about three months ago complained of chest pains. An angiogram revealed that the artery that had the stent was totally blocked. His heart specialist decided that it was not yet a situation requiring further bypass surgery and added diltiazem controlled-release 180 mg tablets daily to the existing medication regimen to control the angina symptoms. Fenofibrate was added to reduce his lipids to more acceptable levels.

Mr. Crockett also suffers from osteoarthritis of the lower back and neck, which is controlled with the meloxicam and glucosamine. His blood pressure has been in the range of 125/70 to 135/85 mmHg since commencing irbesartan some eight years ago.

He is sixty-five years, 5 foot 9 inches (175 cm) tall and weighs 207 pounds (94 kg). His body mass index (BMI) is 30.6 kg/m^2 ($94/1.75^2 =$ or $207/69^2 \times 703 = 30.6$ kg/m^2) placing him just in the obese range).

He lives with his wife and still works some fifty to sixty hours a week in very stressful situations. However, he derives much pleasure from some aspects of his work, despite the fact that some of his employers are putting subtle and not-so-subtle pressure on him to retire. This real or imagined situation causes him great stress and he believes contributes to his deteriorating health. His pathology test results are shown in Table 11.3.

TABLE 11.3. Pathology results for Mr. Crockett over the previous six months.

Physiological value	Six months ago	One month ago	One week ago	Reference values Units	Conventional SI
Potassium	4.2 mEq/L	4.1 mEq/L	4.4 mEq/L	3.5-5 mEq/L	3.5-5.0 mmol/L
Sodium	142 mEq/L	144 mEq/L	143 mEq/L	136-147 mEq/L	136-147 mmol/L
Chloride	102 mEq/L	105 mEq/L	103 mEq/L	95-110 mEq/L	95-110 mmol/L
Bicarbonate	29 mEq/L	27 mEq/L	27 mEq/L	22-31 mEq/L	22-31 mmol/L
Urea	40 mg/dL	49 mg/dL	60 mg/dL	24-49 mg/dL	3-8.2 mmol/L
Creatinine	0.09 mmol/L	0.11 mmol/L	0.14 mmol/L	0.6-1.2 mg/dL	0.05-0.11 mmol/L
Total Cholesterol	260 mg/dL	220 mg/dL	190 mg/dL	<200 mg/dL	<5.2 mmol/L
Triglycerides	220 mg/dL	200 mg/dL	170 mg/dL	<160 mg/dL	<1.8 mmol/L
LDL Cholesterol	145 mg/dL	132 mg/dL	121 mg/dL	<130 mg/dL	<3.36 mmol/L
HDL Cholesterol	38 mg/dL	42 mg/dL	44 mg/dL	>45 mg/dL	>1.16 mmol/L
Chol./HDL ratio	6.8	5.2	4.3		≥ 4.0
Glucose	87 mg/dL	84 mg/dL	85 mg/dL	70-110 mg/dL	3.1-6.1 g/dL
Total protein	7.1 mg/dL	8.0 mg/dL	7.9 mg/dL	6-8 g/dL	60-80 g/L
Albumin	4.3 mg/dL	4 5 mg/dL	4.6 mg/dL	4-6 g/dL	40-60 g/L
Alkaline phosphat	6.5 mg/dL	9.6 mg/dL	18.0 mg/dL	3-12 g/dL	30-120 U/L
Total bilirubin	0.6 mg/dL	0.9 mg/dL	1.1 mg/dL	0.3-1.1 mg/dL	5-19 micromol/L
GGTP	16 U/L	56 U/L	85 U/L	—	<51 U/L
AST (SGOT)	17 U/L	38 U/L	62 U/L	—	≥ 41 U/L
ALT	21 U/L	49 U/L	72 U/L	—	≥ 35U/L
HbA1c	—	—	6.2	—	$\leq 7\%$

Current Medications

Current medications include the following:

- Irbesartan tablets 300 mg qd (for last eight years)
- Atorvastatin tablets 40 mg qd (20 mg d for six years, 40 mg for two years)
- Fenofibrate tablets 160 mg, one daily (introduced four months ago)
- Meloxicam tablets 7.5 mg qd (for last four years)
- Glucosamine 750 mg bid (for last two years)
- Aspirin tablets 100 mg qd (for last eight years)

Diltiazem Extended-release capsules 180 mg qd (introduced two months ago)

Nitroglycerin sublingual tablets 600 mcg prn (never used as he claims to be hypersensitive to them; he tried half a tablet once and almost immediately developed an unbearable headache—is this intelligent noncompliance, or a result of the lack of adequate patient counseling?).

IDENTIFICATION OF DRUG THERAPY PROBLEMS

1. Cardiovascular/cerebrovascular risk factors. Mr. Crockett is at the lower end of obesity; he suffers from significant atherosclerotic disease; he has significant dyslipidemia. His blood pressure is under control with medication. Having already had coronary bypasses, stent, etc.; he is at high risk of a significant metabolic event (heart attack or stroke) (Law, Wald, & Rudnicka, 2003). His physicians have attempted to reduce risk factors with medications.

2. His laboratory test levels show a trend toward increased levels of liver enzymes, urea, and creatinine. The Cockroft-Gault Equation (Hull et al., 1981) is used to calculate creatinine clearance so as to estimate renal function. A slightly modified version (Sansom, 2004) takes into account the ideal body weight of the individual and is shown as follows (for males):

$$\text{Creatinine Clearance (CrCl)mL / min} = \frac{140 - \text{Age(yrs)} \times \text{Ideal Body Weight(Kg)}}{815 \times \text{Serum Creatinine (mmol / L)}}$$

Ideal Body Weight for Males = 50 kg + 0.9 kg/each cm above 152 cm

For Mr. Crockett, Ideal body weight is $= 50 + 0.9 \times (185 - 152) = 79.7$ kg

Therefore, his Creatinine Clearance is $\dfrac{140 - 75 \times 79.7}{815 \times 0.14} = 45.5$ mL / minute

which indicates some level of impairment (normal range of 75 to 125 mL/minute (Koda-Kimble et al., 2005).

POSSIBLE CHANGES IN THERAPY AND BENEFITS/PROBLEMS

Fenofibrate/atorvastatin. The introduction of the fenofibrate to the atorvastatin need careful monitoring as the possibility of myalgias and rhabdomylosis may be additive.

Fenofibrate. The use of the highest dose of the fenofibrate might be inappropriate. An initial dose of 2×67 mg capsules daily based on his creatinine clearance may have been safer; however, the combination seems to have been very effective in lowering Mr. Crockett's C-LDL and triglycerides (USP-DI, 2005).

His biochemical results—dark urine and declared muscle aches and pain as well as his lethargy—could be indicating myolysis with an increased risk of rhabdomyolysis (Pasternak et al., 2002).

Diltiazem and atorvastatin. Diltiazem, has reduced Mr. Crockett's angina symptoms, but may have increased the potential for rhabdomyolysis in that diltiazem inhibits the metabolism of statins (including atorvastatin) via the CYP3A4 isoenzyme pathway, thereby increasing plasma levels of the statin and potential adverse effects (Tatro, 2004).

All these factors combined (high dose atorvastatin + high dose fenofibrate + a CYP3A4 inhibitor + cardiovascular disease + older age + some decreased renal function) significantly increase the risk of Mr. Crockett for developing rhabdomyolysis (Pasternak et al., 2002).

Meloxicam. Meloxicam in a patient with cardiovascular disease should be used with great caution, particularly those with reduced renal function. NSAIDs may reduce the efficacy of antihypertensive agents, as well as potentially increase plasma urea levels (Tatro, 2004); hence the new prescription for 15 mg meloxicam that was prescribed for the muscle pains (myalgia?) may not be appropriate.

POSSIBLE CHANGES IN THERAPY

Arthritis. Until the recent development of aches and pains, his arthritis symptoms were controlled with 7.5 mg meloxicam and glucosamine. Options may include ceasing the long half-life meloxicam with acetaminophen 650 mg to 1000 mg four times a day equivalent; (Semla, Beizer, & Higbee, 2001; Therapeutic Guidelines, 2002) plus a shorter acting NSAID, for example, ibuprofen for breakthrough pain on a prn basis.

Hyperlipidemia. Options for discussion with Mr. Crockett's regular physician are as follows:

1. Reduce dose of fenofibrate to 2×67 mg capsule daily instead of one tablet of 160 mg and continue monitoring lipids, liver enzymes, and creatinine.
2. Consider using ezetimibe 10 mg daily instead of fenofibrate (not as effective in lowering trigycerides as fenofibrate, but less likely to cause myalgias).
3. Possibility of changing atorvastatin to niacin (however, this may not be ideal due to flushing) (Beers, 2000; Koda-Kimble et al., 2005; Sever et al., 2003).
4. Substitute atorvastatin with pravastatin (which is not metabolized via the CYP3A4 pathway (Koda-Kimble et al., 2005; O'Neill et al., 2004). However, this would take some adjustment to reach a level of efficacy that has been obtained with the atorvastatin.

Angina. This is currently reasonably controlled by diltiazem, but it does seem to be causing constipation (Beers, 2000; Koda-Kimble et al., 2005) and possibly contributing to the myalgias (Beers, 2000; Koda-Kimble et al., 2005). Nicorandil, if tolerated by the patient, can be suggested. However, note his stated hypersensitivity to nitroglycerin (Beers, 2000; Koda-Kimble et al., 2005).

Constipation. This may be due to the diltiazem and may be treated with docusate and senna tablets, two at night prn.

Hypertension. This seems to have been under control since he started on the irbesartan. The addition of diltiazem seems to have had no great effect. It might be worth considering a reduction in dose of irbesartan or even deleting it with the addition of the diltiazem.

Outcomes. Development of the medication management plan by the prescriber and Mr. Crockett (after discussion with the pharmacist) resulted in ceasing meloxicam, replacing it with acetaminophen 1 g qid, or a three-times daily dose of a sustained-release preparation if available (to improve adherence), maintaining atorvastatin at 40 mg daily, replacing fenofibrate with ezetimibe 10 mg daily with the physician monitoring Mr. Crockett's symptoms and laboratory values on a monthly basis "until everything settled down." He decided to consider possible use of pravastatin instead of atorvastatin if "things do not settle down." The physician was keen to maintain Mr. Crockett on the diltiazem. He said that the use of nicorandil might be an option "further down the track." At this point in time, he would prefer Mr. Crockett to stay on the irbesartan as well. He agreed that Mr. Crockett should use an aperient on an "as necessary" basis.

Counseling. Mr. Crockett was counseled with respect to diet, such as the frequent eating of fish, a good mixed diet, high fiber and of course a reinforcement of the value of exercise (even walking) in reducing weight and cholesterol levels. Also, it is important that Mr. Crockett sees his physician regularly and has regular blood tests. It should be noted that Mr. Crockett is an extremely well-organized person. He is very keen to do the right thing for his health and is unlikely to be a poor adherer. Reward him with praise to encourage continued compliance, suggest compliance aids, and refill reminders to keep Mr. Crockett on track. Ensure that Mr. Crockett avoids grapefruit and grapefruit juice. This is of particular importance as Mr. Crockett already has a number of agents likely to increase his statin levels.

REFERENCES

ALLHAT Officers and Coordinators for the ALLHAT Collaborative Research Group. (2002). Major outcomes in moderately hypercholesterolemic, hypertensive patients randomized to pravastatin vs usual care: The Antihypertensive and Lipid-Lowering Treatment to Prevent Heart Attack Trial (ALLHAT-LLT). *JAMA, 288:* 2998-3007.

American Heart Association (AHA) (2006a). *Heart disease and stroke statistics—2006 Update.* Dallas, Texas: American Heart Association.

American Heart Association (AHA) (2006b). *High blood cholesterol and other lipids. 2004 update.* Dallas, TX: American Heart Association.

Barraclough, B. (2002). Second national report on patient safety: Improving medication safety Australian Council for Safety & Quality in Health Care, Canberra, Web site.

Beers, M. H. et al. (2000). *The Merck manual of geriatrics* (3rd ed). Section 8, Chapter 63. White House Station, NJ: Merck Research laboratories. Available online: http://www.merck.com/mrkshared/mmg/sec8/sec8.jsp. Accessed September 30, 2006.

CDC National Center for Health Statistics Press (2005). *Deaths; preliminary data for 2003. NVSR, 53*(15): 48.

Dipiro, J. T., Talbert, R. L., Gary, C. Y., et al. (1999). *Pharmacotherapy: A Pathophysiologic Approach* (4th ed.) (pp. 395-418). New York: Appleton & Lange.

Expert panel on the identification, evaluation, and treatment of overweight and obesity in adults (1998). Clinical guidelines on the identification, evaluation, and treatment of overweight and obesity in adults: Executive summary. *Am J Clin Nutr, 68:* 899-917.

Hanlon, J. T., Shimp, L. A., & Semla, T. P. (2000). Recent advances in Geriatrics: Drug-related problems in the elderly. *Ann Pharmacother, 34:* 360-363.

Horowitz, R. I., & Horowitz. S. M. (1993). Compliance to treatment and health outcomes. *Arch Int Med, 153:* 1863-1868.

Hull, J. H., Hak, L. J., Koch, G. G., Wargin, W. A., Chi, S. L., & Mattocks, A. M. (1981). Influence of range of renal function and liver disease on predictability of creatinine clearance. *Clin Pharmacol Ther, 26:* 516-521.

Johnsen, S., Larsson, H., Tarone, R., McLaughlin, J. Nørgård, B., Friis, S., et al. (2005). Risk of hospitalization for myocardial infarction among users of rofecoxib, celecoxib, and other NSAIDs: A population-based case-control study. *Arch Intern Med,* (May 9) *165*(9): 978-984.

Kelley, G. A., Kelley, K. S., & Tran, Z. V. (2004). Walking, lipids, and lipoproteins: A meta-analysis of randomised controlled trials. *Prev Med, 38*(5): 651-661.

Kiortsis, D. N., Giral, P., Bruckert, E., & Turpin, G. (2000). Factors associated with low compliance with lipid-lowering drugs in hyperlipidemic patients. *J Clin Pharm Ther,* (December) *25*(6): 445-451.

Knoops, K., Lisette C., de Groot, L., Kromhout, D., Perrin, A., Moreiras-Varela, O., et al. (2004). Mediterranean diet, lifestyle factors, and 10-year mortality in elderly European men and women: The HALE project. *JAMA, 292*(12): 1433-1439.

Koda-Kimble, M. A., Young, L.Y., Kradjan, W. A., et al. (2005). *Applied Therapeutics: The clinical use of drugs* (8th ed.) (pp. 345-360). Philadelphia: Lippincott Williams & Wilkins.

Law, M. R., Wald, N. J., Morris, J. K., & Jordan, R. E. (2003). Value of low dose combination treatment with blood pressure lowering drugs: Analysis of 354 randomised trials. *BMJ, 326:* 1427-1431.

Law, M. R., Wald, N. J., & Rudnicka, A. R. (2003). Quantifying effect of statins on low density lipoprotein cholesterol, ischaemic heart disease, and stroke: Systematic review and meta-analysis. *BMJ, 326:* 1423-1426.

Lazarou, J., Pomeranz, B. H., & Corey, P. N. (1998). Incidence of adverse drug reactions in hospitalized patients: A meta-analysis of prospective studies. *JAMA* (April 15) *279*(15): 1200-1205.3-8.

Neal, B., MacMahon, S., & Chapman, N. (2000). Blood pressure lowering treatment trialists' collaboration. Effects of ACE inhibitors, calcium antagonists, and other blood-pressure–lowering drugs: Results of prospectively designed overviews of randomised trials. *Lancet, 356:* 1955-1964.

O'Mahony, D., & Martin, U. (1999). *Practical Therapeutics for the Older Patient* (pp. 113-137). Chichester: John Wiley & Sons.

O'Neill, F. H., Brynes, A., Mandeno, R., Rendell, N., Taylor, G., Seed, M., et al. (2004). Comparison of the effects of dietary plant sterol and stanol esters on lipid metabolism. *Nutr Metab Cardiovasc Dis, 14*(3): 133-142.

Pasternak, R. C., Smith, S. C. Jr., Bairey-Merz, C. N., Grundy, S., Cleerman, J., & Lenfant, C. (2002). ACC/AHA/NHLBI clinical advisory on the use and safety of statins. *J Am Coll Cardiol* (August 7) *40*(3): 567-572.

Pignone, M., Phillips, C., & Mulrow, C. (2000). Use of lipid lowering drugs for primary prevention of coronary heart disease: Meta-analysis of randomised trials. *BMJ, 321:* 983-986.

Roller, L., & Gowan, J. (2000). Adherence and the pharmacist. *Australian Journal of Pharmacy, 81*(1): 38-41.

Ross, S., Allen, I., Connelly, J., Korenblat, B., Smith, M., Bishop, D. et al. (1999). Clinical outcomes in statin treatment trials: A meta-analysis. *Arch Intern Med, 159:* 1793-1802.

Roughead, E. E. (1999). The nature and extent of drug-related hospitalisation in Australia. *J Qual Clin Practice, 19:* 19-22.

Sansom, L. N. (2004). *Australian pharmaceutical formulary* (19th ed). Pharmaceutical Society of Australia, Canberra.

Semla, T. P., Beizer, J. L., & Higbee, M. D. (2001). *Geriatric dosage handbook* (6th ed). Cleveland, OH: Lexic-Comps Clinical Reference Library.

Sever, P., Poulter, N., Dahlöf, B., Wedel, H., Collins, R., Beevers, G., et al. (2003). Prevention of coronary and stroke events with atorvastatin in hypertensive patients who have average or lower-than-average cholesterol concentrations, in the Anglo-Scandinavian Cardiac Outcomes Trial–Lipid-Lowering Arm (ASCOT-LLA): A multicentre randomised controlled trial. *Lancet, 361:* 1149-1158.

Simons, L. A., Levis, G., & Simons, J. (1996). Apparent discontinuation rates in patients prescribed lipid-lowering drugs. *Med J Aust, 164:* 208-211.

Simons, L. A., Simons, J., McManus, P., & Dudley, J. (2000). Discontinuation rates for use of statins is high. *BMJ, 321:* 1084.

Tatro, D. S. (2004). *Drug interactions facts, facts & comparisons.* San Carlos: Walters Kluwer Company.

Therapeutic Guidelines: Analgesic Guidelines version 4 (2002). Therapeutic Guideline Limited, Melbourne, Australia.

Thomas, M. C. (2000). Diuretics, ACE inhibitors and NSAIDs—the Triple Whammy. *MJA, 172* (February 21): 184-185.

U.S. Census Bureau Internet Release: Population profile of the United States, 2000. (2003). http://www.census.gov/population/www/pop-profile/profile2000.html.

U.S. Census Bureau 2004, US interim projections by age, sex, race and Hispanic origin. (2005); http://www.gov/ipc/usinterimproj/.

USP DI. (2005. Drug Information for the health care professional (Vol. I) (25th ed.). Thomson MICROMEDEX Greenwood Village, CO.

Wald, N. J., & Law, M. R. (2003). A strategy to reduce cardiovascular disease by more than 80 percent. *BMJ, 326*(7404): 1419-1423.

Chapter 12

Current and Future Considerations

From the previous chapters and contents related to improving compliance, there is a bewildering array of choices pertaining to patient compliance and its improvement. Measurement, enhancement, methods, outcomes, and new models of consideration have all been presented. So, where do we go from here?

ACHIEVING PERFECTION?

After all that has been written here and elsewhere, numerous questions remain, one of which is how much compliance is enough, and are there diminishing returns associated with seeking to achieve 100 percent compliant behavior for patients? The accompanying increase in symptom improvement or decline in illness morbidity for patients may be depicted in Figure 12.1. Does improving compliance lead to a direct correlation with improvement in conditions as depicted by the diagonal line, or is it more reflective of the s-shaped curve? It may vary and be dependent upon patient-, disease-, and drug-related factors. But trying to reach 100 percent as a goal may be unrealistic and unnecessary. Encouraging patients to do their best, and nonjudgmentally evaluating their outcome, along with them, is a better approach to consider.

COMPLICATED CONSIDERATIONS

Figure 12.2 depicts some, but not all, factors that impact compliance, outcomes, and intended and unintended effects. In this depiction, interventions (organizational, educational, behavioral) can lead to

Patient Compliance with Medications: Issues and Opportunities
© 2007 by The Haworth Press, Inc. All rights reserved.
doi:10.1300/5365_12

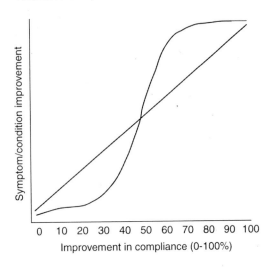

FIGURE 12.1. Diminishing effect of increasing compliance on symptoms or disease.

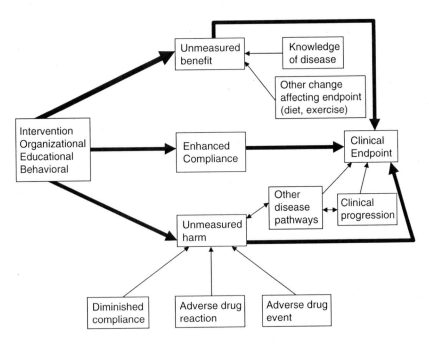

FIGURE 12.2. Compliance and other factors that impact clinical endpoints.

unmeasured benefits, enhanced compliance, or perhaps unmeasured harm. The hoped-for improvement of clinical endpoints may be impacted by interventions improving compliance, but other factors may increase or diminish health effects. Unmeasured harm, adverse effects, lowered levels of compliance, and the impact of other diseases or the progression of diseases can counterbalance the positive effects of interventions leading to affectation of clinical endpoints. Other, unmeasured, positive influences may also impact clinical endpoints that are thought to be improved by compliance. So, unconsidered impact may in fact lead to improvement of endpoints rather than compliance, and so on. Regardless, diminishing complexity cannot surprisingly enhance outcomes.

PHYSICIAN AND DRUG EFFECTS

Misprescribing physicians, or lack of patient knowledge, and adverse drug reactions in combination have devastating effects on patients and compliance (see Figure 12.3). Either can lead to noncompliance and/or lack of efficacy, but instead the patient may be blamed as noted earlier (Lerner, Gulick, & Dubler, 1998). Progress or lack thereof in enhancing physician prescribing, patient knowledge,

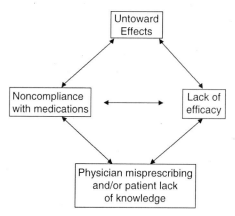

FIGURE 12.3. Interaction of physician and patient variables. *Note:* Physician misprescribing/untoward effects/patient lack of knowledge + decreased efficacy = noncompliance.

or elimination of untoward effects should be shared opportunities between patient, physician, other health providers, and/or caregivers.

Differing Interventions

This author would argue that we need a differentiation of interventions in order to optimally help patients comply with medication regimens. Table 12.1 lists two categories of interventions, catastrophic and wellness. There is overlap of many of the impacts upon compliance namely: personal interaction, organization, education, behavioral packaging, monitoring, follow-up, and concordance. Using a catastrophic identifier to include individual dosing, family and friends, and multiple efforts indicates that additional, intense interventions are necessary. Looking at this another way, one approach is preventive in nature, and one is much more intensive in approach. From what has been written previously in this text, pigeonholing one model, one intervention, or any patient is wrong, but this view of interventions may allow caregivers and patients to understand the importance of interventions and impacts upon noncompliance.

Spectrum of Compliance Outcomes

Figure 12.4 depicts a compliance outcome continuum. In this basic continuum, outcomes can lead to patients being chronically sick or

TABLE 12.1. Compliance interventions.

Catastrophic	Wellness
Personal interaction	Personal interaction
Organization	Organization
Education	Education
Behavioral	Behavioral
Individual Dosing	Packaging
Packaging	Monitoring
Family, friends	Follow-up
Monitoring	Concordance
Follow-up	Preventive
Multiple efforts	
Concordance	

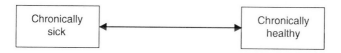

FIGURE 12.4. Spectrum of compliance outcomes.

chronically healthy. Patients may move along this continuum with differing diseases, differing treatments, or advanced age or morbidity. Outcomes may lead to therapeutic effects that are positive or negative, but looking at the issue of compliance outcomes out of the normal approach indicates its importance and relevance.

QUESTIONS (IMPORTANT FACTORS) TO CONSIDER

When anticipating addition or continuation of drug therapies, it would be well for providers to step back and consider the drug and its necessity for treating the patient. Ten questions to ponder when considering patients, current therapies, and additional drugs to be added to the current drugs that the patient is taking are as follows:

1. Is the Drug Needed?

Is a new drug necessary for treatment? Would enhancement of compliance with existing therapies meet the patient/provider needs? Do patients know that a previously prescribed drug can be discontinued with the prescribing of the new agent?

2. Can the Patient Afford the New Drug?

Can the patient afford the prescribed drug? Does the physician know the eventual monetary cost to the patient? Are there less costly alternatives that would provide therapeutic and economic benefit to the patient?—therapeutically in the sense of providing disease or symptom alleviation, and economically by lowering the patient cost and thus helping to ensure initial and continuing compliance. Patients may have fragmented ability to pay for their medications. An example is the effect of Medicare Part D prescription coverage and the associated "donut hole." coverage gap, which may lead to patient noncompliance with therapies (Safran et al., 2005).

3. What Are the Incentives and Trade-Offs for the Patient Benefit-to-Cost Ratio?

What are the benefits of the new drug contrasted with the costs? Here there are many stakeholders who can help to value benefits versus costs. These stakeholders include the patient, physicians, nurses, pharmacists, other health professionals, pharmaceutical manufacturers, the patient's caregivers, the patient's family, programs providing third-party prescription drug coverage (Medicare, Medicaid, etc.). Each of the aforementioned players has a vested interest in the derived answer from comparison of costs and benefits, and the answers may be in conflict with one another. However, patients and the assessment of individual costs and benefits should be the major driver of the "correct" value.

Authors (Giuffrida & Torgerson, 1997) have reviewed studies of paying patients to be compliant with therapies. Ten of eleven studies reviewed by Giuffrida and Torgerson (1997) indicated that financial incentives worked to help patients comply better with drug regimens. There are perhaps other incentives that may be just as, if not, more useful for enhancing compliance. For example, in a similar way that nonsmokers are advantageously provided lower insurance premiums for staying smoke free, can compliant patients with expensive-to-treat illnesses be similarly rewarded for compliant behavior in diabetes, hypertension, congestive heart failure, or other chronic diseases?

4. Are There Predictable Side Effects with the New Therapy?

When drugs are used in real-life patients with other therapies and diseases not seen in clinical trials with narrowly defined patient and therapeutic options, the possibility both of adverse drug events (ADEs) and subsequent noncompliance increases. Has the physician or physicians prescribing for the patient considered all drugs (over-the-counter, prescription, social [caffeine, nicotine, alcohol, drugs of abuse]) that the patient may be consuming? Is the patient prone to ADEs due to disease, demographic, or complexity of therapy regimens?

5. Can the New Drug Take the Place of a Currently Taken Medication?

In the optimal case, the prescribing of a new drug should be accompanied by a subsequent elimination of another drug(s). It may also be very difficult to have this scenario always played out. This add one–eliminate one model may have the most applicability for chronic disease models, but it is an estimable goal. After all the more the drugs prescribed, the more complex the regimen and the more likely the patient noncompliant.

6. Will the New Therapy Lead to the Need to Take More Drugs?

As a corollary to "Can the New Drug Take the Place of a Currently Taken Medication?" does the additional drug added and prescribed lead to the need to further increase the number of drugs taken by patients. Paradoxically and inexplicably (from a commonsense standpoint), pharmaceutical manufacturers actually use this potential coupling of the need for jointly prescribed drugs (as opposed to eliminating a drug) as a potential marketing advantage point. Currently Nexium (esomeprazole magnesium) is being promoted as an adjunct to nonsteroidal or coxx-2 inhibitor therapies in order to solely reduce gastrointestinal (GI) complications of pain-relief medication use. The use of Nexium is promoted as a sensible approach to reducing GI effects.

Currently advertisements are appearing on television, and duplicated on the Internet website (http://www.purplepill.com), that depict an elderly couple on their living room couch discussing the wife's need to take Nexium to reduce GI effects occurring with her use of analgesic agents. Could, as an alternative, the patient try using acetaminophen and discontinue the NSAID therapy and the need to subsequently take an agent to decrease NSAID induced gastropathy?

7. Has the Patient "Bought into" the Need for the New Drug, for example, Use of Concordance?

Is the dynamic relationship between physicians and patients such that the patient is encouraged and empowered to move past a pacifist to an activist role relative to their care? Is there a linguistic mismatch between patient and provider? Is the patient sufficiently health literate to understand and assimilate the physician-directed questions, instructions, and/or treatment plan?

The concordance model is a method worth emulating to improve the dynamic between patient and physician. To drill down here, has the patient been brought into the decision-making process concerning the drugs prescribed? We need to move away from therapy "silos" where physician and patient exist in a mutually exclusive environment. There is a need to adequately interact to ensure patient buy-in and tie-in. Personal health records and health information technology advancements need to incorporate patient accessibility and input into future system architecture.

Can Compliance Be Monitored?

Health care technology has advanced to such a degree that patients can be monitored electronically to assess compliance (e.g., container, computers, other electronic recorders). Yet our software and electronic capabilities are not being brought to bear on the pandemic of patient noncompliance. We need to move past a paper- and person-driven process of monitoring care to a system where caregivers and patients can use technology to enhance compliance behavior.

8. Is the New Drug Being Prescribed to Pacify the Patient?

Is the drug being prescribed really necessary for the patient? Does the prescribing of the drug serve nontherapeutic purposes? In other words, does the drug prescribing conveniently end the physician–patient encounter resulting in an unnecessary drug being prescribed (Bisno, 2001) rather than helping to meet patient–physician goals in treatment and outcomes? Physicians may be gaming the system by using a prescribed drug to end the patient encounter and pacify patients. The convenient writing of a new prescription in order to meet nontherapeutic needs that are not drug related may help the physician avoid a bothersome patient encounter or confrontation, end the patient encounter in a short visit, and thus eliminate the need to spend additional time with the patient.

9. Have Nondrug Alternatives Been Tried First Before Prescribing Drug?

Is it more important to use a drug or can a nondrug alternative (diet, exercise, behavior) meet both physician and patient needs? Can the patient be given incentives to be intelligently noncompliant to substitute a behavioral, nutrition, diet, and/or exercise therapy as opposed to taking a new drug that might not work as well as a nondrug alternative? Could mild hypertension, obesity, diabetes, or other condition be treated by a nondrug so as to avoid increasing medication regimen complexity by adding more and more drugs to be consumed?

10. Will Food–Drug, Drug–Diet, or Drug–Drug Interactions Be Likely with the New Drug and Currently Consumed Medications?

Many drugs have predictable and serious drug interactions associated with their use initially and perhaps in the long term. The need is to adequately consider both the potential for drug interactions to occur, and to contemplate the substitution of drugs that may be less likely to instigate interactions with other drugs, foods, or consumed items.

FUTURE CONSIDERATIONS WITH EMERGING DRUG THERAPIES

Pharmacogenomics provides a tantalizing view of the future, both therapeutically and economically. The use of single pharmaogenomic agents to avoid the use of multiple therapies can provide significant, positive, outcomes for both therapeutic and cost considerations. However, the costs of new therapies will not come in inexpensive therapies. The ability of patients to pay coupled with the potential for enhanced compliance with less challenging compliance regimens will be difficult decisions for patient, caregivers, and providers to make.

Shaffer (2004b), in analyzing beneficial aspects of new pharmacogenomically derived products for treatment of HIV, points to several positive advantages of the new and emerging therapies. Currently, treatment for HIV AIDS is both costly and exceedingly complex to comply with. At present, the predominant treatment regime for HIV, called HAART for Highly Active Anti-Retroviral Therapy, is complex and challenging to comply with. A new agent, pharmacogenomically derived, PA-457, targets the final step of viral infection, when the virus is released from the cell. Emerging therapy with one agent can be used to remove the need to take multiple therapies at multiple times during the day. These new therapies may, however, be accompanied attendant exorbitant costs.

Terry (2004) notes the promise of pharmacogenomics in reducing both side effects and diminishing problems with patient noncompliance. Terry notes that side effects with oral administration of drugs may be substantially reduced and both acceptance and patient compliance improved for patients. However, intravenous or other parenteral drug therapy administration needs may also stress patient compliance and acceptance. The paradox is that the new agents may be less complex to comply with, but be more challenging to adequately administer due to parenteral, storage, and administration requirements. The less complex dosing intervals may be offset by increasing complexity of administration requirements. Terry (2004) presents transdermal delivery devices that provide access to complex proteins that are the product of pharmacogenomic research. Use of the transdermal approach to administer drugs would eliminate the hassles associated with patient self-administration of parenteral therapies.

Shaffer (2004a) notes that a highly selective protein for use in treating Alzheimer's disease and Parkinson's syndrome has selective properties. Shaffer optimistically points that this new therapy in clinical trials at present bypasses current dilemmas related to compliance with currently available pharmacotherapies for neurological conditions. Patients with these conditions will no doubt continue to require caregiver assistance in order to achieve therapeutic and compliance outcomes that are beneficial. Parenteral drug administration requirements will add stress to patient ability to self-administer these drugs, and require caregiver assistance.

Class (2004) argues for the pharmacogenomically derived designer drugs as being drugs worth paying for therapeutic and economic reasons. Targeted cures, enhanced compliance, and positive cost-benefit ratio assessments highlight the appropriateness of payment for pharmacogenomically derived pharmaceuticals. The ushering in of personalized medicine will help patients, providers, and certainly manufacturers seeking top-dollar reimbursement for research and development, and marketing costs.

Counterbalancing of the promise of these new therapies, with the realization of administration concerns related to compliance, will be a task necessary to complete for patients, providers, caregivers, and policy decision makers.

Medicare Part D Outpatient Drug Therapy Coverage

Beginning in 2006, Medicare through Part D began payment for outpatient drug therapies for Medicare recipients who signed up for coverage. This important and revolutionary change in payment for outpatient drug therapies for seniors will be interesting to observe, monitor, and measure outcomes for the near and long-term future. Patients will be provided drug therapies within the program, and the amount will vary as depicted in Table 12.2. After a deductible amount is reached patients will receive benefits up to a certain level and then have a period of non-coverage through Part D. For the majority of patients spending between $2,250 and $5,100, there will be no coverage in 2006.

TABLE 12.2. Medicare Part D coverage, deductibles, and gaps for patients.

Patient drug costs	Patients to pay	Medicare pays	Patient total out-of-pocket costs per year*
$0-$250	100% ($250)	$0	$250
$251-$2,250	25% ($500)	75% ($1,500)	$750
$2,251-$5,100	100% ($2850)	$0	$3,600
Over $5,100	5%	95%	$3,600 + 5% of costs above $5,100

Note: *Does not include premium costs.

And after $5,100 is spent a 5 percent co-payment is required after that point.

How this will affect patient compliance will be individual and variable. Many seniors struggle as it is with compliance, and factoring in the variable cost of drugs may impact many patients in a negative manner relative to compliance. As can be seen in Table 12.2, the co-payment, coinsurance, and deductible amounts will increase rather steadily over the next decade. This increase coupled with increasing monthly premiums will tax many seniors and again variously impact their drug-taking compliance behavior. Cubanski and colleagues (2005) recently reported the impact of increasing numbers of drugs, and variable payment mechanisms excluding coverage as having a negative influence on patient compliance. Regardless, the outcomes and behaviors (both patient and provider) will be rich, empirical, areas for drug-related research in the future.

WHERE DO WE GO FROM HERE?

We cannot continue to accept the unacceptable. Punitive reactions to patients, inappropriate blaming of the patient for noncompliance, and increased prescribing of new drugs despite previous problems with patients' compliance activities need to be halted and another view of patient care to be implemented. The concordance model is a fine place to start, but continuing and personalized attention to patients and patients' needs require to be much more of an accepted activity rather than the occasional reaction to patient noncompliance.

REFERENCES

Bisno, A. L. (2001). Acute pharyngitis. *NEJM, 344*(3): 205-211.

Class, S. (2004). Personalised medicine: Quality not quantity. IMS Global Insights. Accessed on August 8, 2005 at: http://www.imshealth.com/web/content/0,3148, 64576068_63872702_70515404_70684915,00.html.

Cubanski, J., Voris, M., Kitchman, M., Neuman, T., & Potetz, L. (2005). *Medicare chartbook* (3rd ed.). Washington, DC: The Henry J. Kaiser Family Foundation.

Giuffrida, A., & Torgerson, D. J. (1997). Should we pay the patient? Review of financial incentives to enhance patient compliance. *BMJ, 315:* 703-707.

Lerner, B. H., Gulick, R. M., & Dubler, N. N. (1998). Rethinking nonadherence, historical perspectives on triple-drug therapy for HIV Disease. *Annals of Internal Medicine, 129*(7): 573-578.

Safran, D. G., Neuman, P., Schoen, C., Kitchman, M. S., Wilson, I. B., Cooper, B., Li, A., Chaing, H., & Rogers, W. H. (2005). Prescription drug coverage and seniors: Findings from a 2005 national survey. *Health Aff* (April 1): W5-152-W5-166.

Shaffer, C. (2004a). Chaperone protein dissolves amyloid plaques. *Genomics & Proteomics.* 5/02/04. Accessed August 9, 2005 at www.genpromag.com.

Shaffer, C. (2004b). New anti-HIV compound inhibits virus maturation. *Genomics & Proteomics.* 7/02/04. Accessed August 9, 2005 at www.genpromag.com.

Terry, M. (2004). Dermatrends announces patent for amine drug delivery system. *Genomics & Proteomics.* 07/06/0404. Accessed August 9, 2005 at www.genpromag.com.

Index

Page numbers followed by the letter "f" indicate figures; those followed by the letter "t" indicate tables.

Patient Compliance with Medications: Issues and Opportunities
© 2007 by The Haworth Press, Inc. All rights reserved.
doi:10.1300/5365_13

Order a copy of this book with this form or online at:
http://www.haworthpress.com/store/product.asp?sku=5365

PATIENT COMPLIANCE WITH MEDICATIONS
Issues and Opportunities

_____ in hardbound at $59.95 (ISBN: 978-0-7890-2609-5)

_____ in softbound at $32.95 (ISBN: 978-0-7890-2610-1)

208 pages plus index • Includes illustrations

Or order online and use special offer code HEC25 in the shopping cart.

COST OF BOOKS_____

☐ **BILL ME LATER:** (Bill-me option is good on US/Canada/Mexico orders only; not good to jobbers, wholesalers, or subscription agencies.)

POSTAGE & HANDLING_____
(US: $4.00 for first book & $1.50 for each additional book)
(Outside US: $5.00 for first book & $2.00 for each additional book)

☐ Check here if billing address is different from shipping address and attach purchase order and billing address information.

Signature_____

SUBTOTAL_____

☐ **PAYMENT ENCLOSED:** $_____

IN CANADA: ADD 6% GST_____

☐ **PLEASE CHARGE TO MY CREDIT CARD.**

STATE TAX_____
(NJ, NY, OH, MN, CA, IL, IN, PA, & SD residents, add appropriate local sales tax)

☐ Visa ☐ MasterCard ☐ AmEx ☐ Discover
☐ Diner's Club ☐ Eurocard ☐ JCB

Account # _____

FINAL TOTAL_____
(If paying in Canadian funds, convert using the current exchange rate, UNESCO coupons welcome)

Exp. Date_____

Signature_____

Prices in US dollars and subject to change without notice.

NAME_____

INSTITUTION_____

ADDRESS_____

CITY_____

STATE/ZIP_____

COUNTRY_____ COUNTY (NY residents only)_____

TEL_____ FAX_____

E-MAIL_____

May we use your e-mail address for confirmations and other types of information? ☐ Yes ☐ No
We appreciate receiving your e-mail address and fax number. Haworth would like to e-mail or fax special discount offers to you, as a preferred customer. **We will never share, rent, or exchange your e-mail address or fax number.** We regard such actions as an invasion of your privacy.

Order From Your Local Bookstore or Directly From
The Haworth Press, Inc.
10 Alice Street, Binghamton, New York 13904-1580 • USA
TELEPHONE: 1-800-HAWORTH (1-800-429-6784) / Outside US/Canada: (607) 722-5857
FAX: 1-800-895-0582 / Outside US/Canada: (607) 771-0012
E-mail to: orders@haworthpress.com

For orders outside US and Canada, you may wish to order through your local
sales representative, distributor, or bookseller.
For information, see http://haworthpress.com/distributors

(Discounts are available for individual orders in US and Canada only, not booksellers/distributors.)

PLEASE PHOTOCOPY THIS FORM FOR YOUR PERSONAL USE.
http://www.HaworthPress.com   BOF07

Dear Customer:

Please fill out & return this form to receive special deals & publishing opportunities for you! These include:

- availability of new books in your local bookstore or online
- one-time prepublication discounts
- free or heavily discounted related titles
- free samples of related Haworth Press periodicals
- publishing opportunities in our periodicals or Book Division

❑ OK! Please keep me on your regular mailing list and/or e-mailing list for new announcements!

Name _____

Address_____

STAPLE OR TAPE YOUR BUSINESS CARD HERE!

_____

*E-mail address _____

*Your e-mail address will never be rented, shared, exchanged, sold, or divested. You may "opt-out" at any time. May we use your e-mail address for confirmations and other types of information? ❑ Yes ❑ No

Special needs:
Describe below any special information you would like:

- Forthcoming professional/textbooks
- New popular books
- Publishing opportunities in academic periodicals
- Free samples of periodicals in my area(s)

Special needs/Special areas of interest:

_____

_____

_____

_____

Please contact me as soon as possible. I have a special requirement/project:

_____

_____

_____

_____

The Haworth Press Inc.

PLEASE COMPLETE THE FORM ABOVE AND MAIL TO:
Donna Barnes, Marketing Dept., The Haworth Press, Inc.
10 Alice Street, Binghamton, NY 13904–1580 USA
Tel: 1–800–429–6784 • Outside US/Canada Tel: (607) 722–5857
Fax: 1–800–895–0582 • Outside US/Canada Fax: (607) 771–0012
E-mail: orders@HaworthPress.com

GBIC07